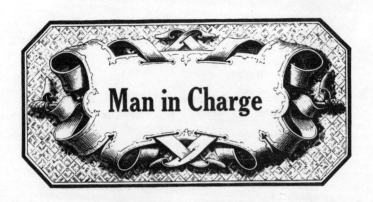

Man in Charge

The Executive's Guide
to Grooming, Manners, and Travel

John Weitz

Macmillan Publishing Co., Inc.
New York

Library of Congress Cataloging in Publication Data

Weitz, John.
  Man in charge.

  1. Grooming for men. 2. Men's clothing.
3. Business etiquette. 4. Voyages and travels—
1951-
—Guides-books. I. Title.
RA777.8.W44   646.7'02'4041   74-11214
ISBN 0-02-625770-X

Macmillan Publishing Co., Inc.
866 Third Avenue, New York, N. Y. 10022
Collier-Macmillan Canada Ltd.

First Printing 1974

Printed in the United States of America

To my friend, collaborator, and editor, EVERETT MATTLIN, all my sincere thanks. While this book was being written, he was my sounding board, my pepper-upper, my calmer-downer, and he soundly believed in the fun and value of this project.

———————◆•◆———————

This book is also for P. and C.,
who will surely be M.I.C.

Table of Contents

The First Word

Holy Harvard Business School. And Wharton. And M.I.T. Was there ever a man like America's businessman? Bright, sharp, driving, alert, creative, thrusting . . . and, in some ways, *dumb as hell*.

What else can you call a guy who can be hard-nosed in his office and yet will be conned by hair-dressers and haberdashers. A super business planner who clutters up his everyday personal existence. A handsome fellow who ruins his own looks. A corporate vice-president who cringes before head-waiters. A warm, friendly guy who can manage to seem pompous and arrogant. A mature, experienced man who tries to imitate some half-assed kids.

The funny part is that he's often bright enough to *know* that somewhere he's going wrong, that somehow something grates. Nothing big, mind you, nothing major, just the feeling that some other guys seem to live more smoothly, with more style.

I wrote this book to help this man who feels slightly uneasy. And to help his wife who grabbed me at a party and whispered, "Can't you get Marvin to cut off those stupid fat sideburns? After all it makes him look so *bald* on top and he's only 50."

Dear lady, I'll try.

(Just between you and me and the computer, Marvin's really 52.)

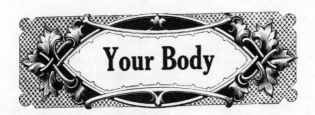

Your Body

Taking Care of the Basics

The Face

That poor, poor face. I mean, how would *you* like to wake up day after day to confront cold steel?

No wonder most men's faces look like moonscapes by the time they're forty.

Yes, I know you've been shaving since you were sixteen and you're no longer sixteen and you know what's best for you. *But . . .*

Why don't we review the daily shave and consider how you can make things easier for your puss. To begin with, wash your face with hot water and soap. Nothing at all to do with cleanliness, but everything to do with softening your bristles. Most shave creams, all by themselves, haven't the muscle. Then rinse off the soap, again with hot water, hot as you can take it without turning crimson. Leave the water and spread on shave cream. Then wait a little while, just enough to inspect the bags under your eyes and throw a devil-may-care smirk at yourself—say a count of ten or fifteen.

Then start shaving, *and shave only with the grain.* If your blade is sharp, you'll be clean enough. Shaving against the grain is terribly rough on your hide. I know the barbers do it, but they have a deft touch. You're a ham fist. We all are. If your blade isn't sharp enough, get another blade.

It's cheaper to buy new blades—and the best in the
drugstore—than a new face. If your new blade
won't do, change blade brands or change razors.

Anyway, most of us look clean after one good
with-the-grain shave and to go beyond that is pure
paranoia. Didn't know you could be paranoid
about your stubble, did you? Part of it comes from
those years of viewing advertising about five
o'clock shadow and the nubs, while the remainder
lies deeper within you—somewhere in the tur-
moiled recesses of your insecure psyche. But it
hardly warrants treatment. I mean, how can you
lie down on the couch and begin with, "Doc, you
see, all day long I go around feeling that people
are staring at me because I am not, er, clean-
shaven. . . ."

Lastly, after you've gotten rid of one-way stubble and soap flecks, try this: Use a sun cream, like
Bain de Soleil (the bronze kind which gives you a
gratuitous tennis tan), and massage it into your
face, forehead, eyelids, bags under eyes, cheeks,
and aggressive chin (and any other chins you are
called on to maintain). Somehow, because the sun
creams all contain good stuff like lanolin, it helps.
All the elasticity comes back after your bout with
the steel, and the cream even seems to iron out the
wrinkles a bit.

Now get into the shower, but don't soap your
face. Plain water will wash off some of the sun
cream, leaving enough to let you face the world.

A few very private reminders. (Prissy males
may skip this section, and female readers should
not read it unless they shave their faces each morning, in which case, the whole damn book may be
of interest to them.)

Hair in nose. Clip it. Carefully. There are

special nose scissors with safety tips made. It is important. You know what I mean.

Hair in ears. Most barbers, if they're friends, will do the trimming for you. Don't try it yourself. Unless you're van Gogh.

Hair next to nose. There are some stubborn hairs which are out of reach of your razor and which grow like mad. They look like hell. Get some tweezers and eradicate them. Out. By the roots. You must be ruthless.

Cold weather lips. Use anti-chap stick. Also, try to stop licking your lips at zero-degree temperatures. That's how they chap in the first place. The way to use anti-chap stick is *not* to hold it in your fingertips like a lady touching up her mouth after necking. Rather, hold it in your fist like a tennis racket. It will make a better impression should someone see you.

A quick note for those of you who are occasional guests on TV. Makeup men are *not* in your corner. For instance: you arrive looking nice and tanned and healthy and the makeup Rembrandt says, "Tsk . . . we'll have to eliminate that beard." Then he powders you stone white. The real reason he is pasting your face is that *you* look great and the *host* of the show looks like hell; they're powdering you down to look more haggard than the star. You no like? Say so. Say *no*.

The Sun Lamp

Most metropolitan business types spend their winters in pale-faced fatigue. You may line up five traveling days with lots of meetings and lots of late nights and come home looking like you've been interrogated by the Gestapo.

There are two solutions. One is to rush away to the sunshine each weekend. But time is money, and even if you had the time, you still might not have the money.

The other is a *sun lamp*.

Used with gentle care, it can give you a deceptively healthy look. They have the fold-up kind for travel, too. Here's how to hype up your appearance:

Apply some good sun lotion right after you shave. Then use the sun lamp—forty-five seconds on the right, a minute in the front and forty-five seconds on the left side of your face. Cover your eyes, of course, dummy! Within a few days you'll look like the brawny, spunky devil you think you are.

The payoff comes when you look at yourself in the mirror. Reflected back is that bronzed hero of your fantasies.

Never mind about the rest of you. People only

judge by your face. They can't tell you're milky white on the left buttock.

Serious note: If you've ever had skin troubles of any kind, check with your doctor before you embark on the sun-lamp routine. Otherwise, or if your doctor says okay, go to it.

Hair

Historically, in the context of Western civilization—and recent years haven't contradicted this—long hair has meant the disorganized man: the poet, the romantic, the philosopher, the rebel, the prophet, the holy man.

Conversely, short hair has meant decisiveness, aggressiveness, cleanliness, athletic agility, directness, and precision.

Now have a look at all the above qualities and apply them to your own life—*ignoring any pressures to conform to the "latest" thing.* (Why should you conform, anyway?)

For instance. You're an accountant, a cracker-jack accountant. What is your best image? Should you look vague, dreamy, mystical? Or should you look forceful, direct, and organized? The answer is clear.

Yet . . . many accountants around you these days are growing sideburns, Fu Manchu moustaches, and curly hair in back (it's tough to do on top when hair just ain't there). Besides, your wife needles you to break out and the kids needle you to get with it and you're already too scared to face your barber because it's been five weeks since you last saw him. Then, too, you're a man of the times, aren't you? and therefore a part of the men's fashion revolution.

Like hell you are! You're a crackerjack accountant *who needs a haircut*, that's what you are. Deep in your soul you know it already. All that floppy gray hair makes you feel messy. Every time the wind hits you, it's all over your head and you're ashamed to go into a serious meeting without a careful combing session. You wish you had a haircut just so you could *know* you look neat.

Neat. That's what you're *supposed* to be, professionally. Neat brain, neat figures, neat facts, neat appearance. Doctors should have clean fingernails and politicians should wear sincere ties and accountants should be neat. Even $150,000-a-year accountants.

Let's go on from there (even if it may hurt). You're a very senior executive in a company which hasn't been doing so hot lately. You're about to go into a board meeting to explain to the directors why things haven't been so good and why you don't expect to set the world on fire in the next six months either. Should you look romantic? Poetic? Not if you want to keep that office with the Bigelow on the floor, you shouldn't.

Or: You're rather discouraged because some of the people in your division, some of your brightest lights, haven't been burning the midnight fluorescent. These, your prize protégés, have been letting you down. Admit it. Their weekends start Thursday evening and end Monday afternoon. Oh, they're at their desks physically all right, but they might as well be back in the sack with their weekend dates. You've read *Up the Organization*, and you're sure that you've "created the proper climate" and all, but they just ain't producing.

Could it be that you've been misleading them with your own flamboyance? Maybe the length of your hair or sideburns isn't the measure of your own hard-work input, but to a younger member of the organization, who is bound to take his cue from you, it may give false signals. You buy a Ferrari, he'll buy an M.G. You seem devil-may-care, he'll feel "I don't give a damn."

Finally, one supreme brutality. Long hair is youthful. Loose hair is youthful. Your face will suffer by contrast. One of those stylist-created, exquisitely wavy, loose, casual hairdos atop bushy sideburns on a craggy middle-aged face *can add years and years to your appearance*! I know, you thought it was the opposite, but take another look at some of those middle-aged executive bushmen. Cropping those locks would crops years off their physiognomies.

A short, neat, casual haircut (without any high-polish sleekness) is bound to show those hard-earned wrinkles in the best light. You'll look experienced and wise, tough (but with a heart of gold), like an old salt or an airlines captain, or a guy who climbed Everest twenty years back.

Hair Dyeing

There is a crucial moment when every man searches his mirror and then searches his soul. It occurs around the age of thirty-five.

Hey, am I getting grey? Around the temples, maybe. Or in streaks. Or all-over salt and pepper.

If the mirror's answer is an unmistakable *yes*, then comes the soul-searching. Should I hit the bottle? Dye, that is, not Scotch (though you may need a shot of the latter at this point).

If you have started to *lose* your hair, put the option of dyeing out of your mind. Your eventual problem is not going to be the color of your hair, but the gloss of your skin. It doesn't matter a hoot if a balding man has grey hair or red hair around the fringes. People will see what's not there, not what is. A slim, young face will help. Nothing else will—except a hairpiece, of course, which is a whole 'nother chapter.

But if you have a full head of strong hair, you have a decision to make. If you fancy the image of "prematurely grey with very young face and fine figure," then by all means forget hair dyes and concentrate on the calorie counting and the gym workouts.

If you are gaining a slight paunch, however,

you can decide to touch up *slightly*. It will then be possible to be somewhat chubby while still looking quite young.

The business of really dyeing your hair, of making a radical transformation from grey to total dark brown, is usually disastrous. No matter how good the dyestuff and how skillful the ministrations of Pierre, they are somehow never quite good enough. Everyone around you knows you didn't turn auburn-haired overnight. Most important, *you* know you didn't, at least naturally. The awareness that you are dyeing your hair imposes a new sense of insecurity—and that, chum, is the last thing anyone needs.

The big choice comes when you approach thirty-five, as I said. Once you've rounded forty, forget the whole thing. You've been around too long. No one will believe you. You won't even believe yourself. You'll *know* you look fake.

Toupee or Not Toupee

At first it's the suspicion that all is not well on top. Perhaps it's the barber whom you catch shaking his head. ("What's wrong, Mario? Am I getting thin on top?" "Of *course* not! You? Thin on top? You've got enough hair for fifty years to come. . . .") Or maybe you catch a glint of scalp in the two-way mirror when you're having a suit fitted. Or maybe your wife strokes your hair and suddenly her fingers seem very cold.

Whatever, you have to face it: you're losing some top-stuff. Your comb becomes your enemy—a shark which comes away with mouthfuls of hair. You can't believe it. You, who had those long wavy locks. You, who had to use greasy kids' stuff back there in college to get that shock of thick, luxurious growth to behave.

And you're depressed. Christ, you're depressed. A cold grey dawn, a bleak terrain, a suspicion that you have passed your peak and are sliding. For a while you still don't quite believe it. You recomb your hair in different ways. You push your fingers through it often, to check up. You keep telling yourself that the terrible recession is over.

Then you bump into Al. Al is an old friend whom you see rarely, which is lucky, because Al presumes upon the longevity of your friendship to be unkindly blunt. He's the guy with the "Hey, you've put on a little, haven't you?" chuckle, chuckle, pat-on-your-belly. He's the one who winks and gives you the (whistle) "Great secretary you took to that convention in Omaha. . . ." And *he's* the one who is bound to say "Hi, skinhead . . ." or something equally jolly.

And one day you are bald. Just like that. It often happens quickly. One or two years. Now what? Hara-kiri? The Shrink? The Toupee Maker?

About toupees. They are fantastic. There is no doubt that the modern toupee is almost undetectable. I can't knock it. And perhaps no one knows you're wearing one, except you and your wife and your kids and your secretary and everyone else who's been around you in the last twenty years. So who are you kidding? Strangers? If it's romance you're after, you'll live in mortal fear of the moment when it's tangle-time and your wig gets dislodged. Better business impression? Makes you look younger? Perhaps. On the other hand, *hardly* anyone can detect your wig, but *someone* might, and so you'll always feel on the defensive.

It's true that movie actors wear them successfully on screen. But the screen is another matter. After all, they also wear desert-dust makeup when they ride on a horse and false moustaches and body makeup for gladiator scenes. The screen is make-believe and the viewer is removed from the wig-wearer by lighting and photography and atmosphere *and his own willingness to believe in the character on screen.*

But real life is not a Warner Brothers production.

(Even screen actors face penalties for their

make-believe. Do you know how it feels to grab a machine gun and run past fake explosions through fake battles and fake bullets, shooting blank cartridges? *With a whole crew of tough movie grips and prop men watching*? Some of the old timers, the John Waynes, don't give a hoot anymore. But a few of them—and many of the newer screen rowdies—spend a lot of off-screen time proving to themselves and all the industry that they are indeed tough guys—out of sheer embarrassment.)

Anyway, I'm not telling you *not* to wear a toupee. But I *am* telling you that it's best to be yourself. If you're bald, then be bald. Believe me, if you're a charming, amusing guy, no one, man or woman, will penalize you for baldness.

Hands

You wave them around in front of people. They're always on display. They should look good.

Manicurists are dear girls. They're chatty and they know the gossip and they're attractive in a manicurist sort of way. But are they *always* necessary? Okay, if you've been off on a hunting trip or painting the bottom of your boat or giving your awl to a do-it-yourself kick in the basement, your nails may be mangled. Then, rush to the manicurist. With one proviso: don't allow her to buff your nails to make them shiny. It smacks of cardsharp and waxed moustachios.

Most of the time, though, you can take care of your own hands. Just be sure your nails are clipped and clean. Keep them neatly cut and filed, and then *brush* under the nails with a stiff brush, morning and night and, if possible, in between. Don't use the tips of steel files to gouge under your nails. The undersides will get scraped and scratched and catch more dirt more quickly.

If you've been working on the car ("just puttering with the old Bentley") or checking out the engine room of your palatial yacht, use the kind of grease soap the mechanics use or a strong detergent.

The main thing is clean, clean, clean.

Now, about rings on those fingers.

Most married blokes should wear wedding bands. You're married—period. Doesn't matter if it ruins an airplane romance. (Sooner or later you'll have to tell her you're married, anyway.) But once you wear a wedding band, it's tough to wear another ring on the same hand. Maybe on the other. If your left hand's banded and you are super wild about your family crest or your Annapolis past, wear the thing on the right hand.

Some men, with *large* hands, can wear pinky signet rings. With small hands, the ring overwhelms the hand.

Diamond rings for men are *out*. Hear me? O-U-T! They're a hangover from the gambling twenties. You're secure now. Safe now. You don't have to hock a ring anymore. Or if you do, hock your *wife's*.

About wedding bands: the nice, square, old wedding ring is . . . well . . . nice and square and old. Why not switch to a wide masculine band or to a very thin band? Make it a grand shebang, a rewedding ceremony. Go on a second honeymoon.

Rings on the thumb, index finger, or middle finger are not for grown men. Not since Henry the Eighth.

Ring wearer, please remember that other men wear rings too, and that you can mangle their claws if your rings catch theirs when you shake hands and squeeze. Have you ever seen a grown man with tears in his eyes saying "How d'y'do?"

You should shake hands *firmly*, to show you're a straightforward, honorable, dear, warm, hearty peach of a guy. But there's a difference between firmly and viciously. There's even a difference between vigorously and viciously. Beware the vicious handshaker. Or close the car door on his drinking hand at some opportune moment. It'll ease the squeeze.

Hands can be hooked into vest pockets, galluses or vest armholes. It's a quaint, old-fashioned, Justice Holmes sort of gesture. It also makes you look like a pompous ass. Don't clutch your lapels either. It's the same syndrome. It also bends the lapels.

And a final touchy subject, just between us. Very private.

When driving in your car, all by yourself, deep in thought, don't investigate the inside of your nose. Thousands of grown men do it. Unfortunately, the people in the next car see it, and with your luck it'll be your oldest daughter's newest boyfriend whom you've lambasted about pot. He'll blackmail you.

The Shower, The Bath

To most people the shower is just . . . a shower. To those who *know*, it's an adventure.

Consider. You can tune it cool to begin with, then heat it up, then back down to cool. You can, of course, sing. You can do Weitz' favorite tummy exercise (see below).

You can experiment. For instance, if you're really beat and hot and drooping at the end of a summer day, try this: Turn your shower to *luke-warm*, just a touch of warmth, and then turn your back to it, letting the stream run over your neck and down your back and chest. I promise you— *Nirvana*!

One thing. You *must* stick your head under the water, else a shower is no good. You should feel as if you've been for a swim in the pool, and anyway it's good for your hair to get wet, to get the surface dust out. Any hairdo you can't stick under the shower is *useless*.

But if you really want to pamper the old frame, try a *bath*. Oh, I know, you haven't used the tub for years. Showers, showers, showers. Rush, rush, rush. Women take baths, right? Wrong.

Most of us are forced into baths when we go to Europe, because most European showers are

odd things on the end of flexible hoses, like tele-
phones. And they have about as much force as an
elder gent suffering with prostatitis. But once you
rediscover the occasional bath ("Haven't taken one
since I was a kid"), you'll bless me.

And use all sorts of pampering gimmicks. Like
pouring some of your after-shave or cologne into
the water before you climb in. Steal some of "her"
bubble bath. Read the evening paper. Or the morning paper. Or have a cup of coffee. Or a martini.
Or just listen to the local FM station. Examine
your toenails. (Need clipping?) Buy one of those
bath rests and bath tables so you can settle in.

Then take a shower. Whee!

My favorite tummy exercise:
Breathe out completely. Then tuck in your
tummy as if you were trying to touch your spine
with it. Hold it six seconds. Then let your tummy
out and take a deep breath. Huff. Puff. Huff. Puff.
You're in good shape, eh?

Repeat the whole thing three more times.
Then the fourth time, hold your breath and tuck
your tummy in for ten seconds.

Then collapse.

It tones up the flab.

It's isometric.

That's isometric?

Yes, Arthur, that's isometric.

I give no guarantees about instant waist loss.
This is for tone, not tonnage. But look at it this
way: What've I got to lose? It's cheap and fast.
And I know a guy who swears he went from 36" to
34" in three weeks. Of course, he also stopped
boozing.

Before you do the above daring thing ask your

doc if it's okay. If he says you shouldn't tuck in your tummy or hold your breath, of course, don't. But you'd better see the nurse on the way out and make a date for a checkup.

Walking Right, Sitting Right... and Moving Right

You can walk "fat." You can sit "fat." You can even scratch yourself "fat." You can also walk "old" and sit "old" and scratch yourself . . . well, you can.

There are just endless postural, gestural ways of letting yourself down while being completely unaware of it. Look at John Wayne. There he is, post-cancer-operation, post-sixty, and overweight. Yet he walks and sits and moves like a young'un and the dames are still mad about him. Or look at Gable, there toward the very end, in the *Misfits*, when he was well over fifty and pretty worn down. He *moved* right. And Flynn (Erroll, of course), when he was in boozy maturity; and Cagney and Astaire and Doug Fairbanks, Jr. and Walter Pidgeon. All of them knew the secret. How to *move*.

First, you have to imagine that you're back in your springy youth. Go ahead, try to remember what it felt like. Remember the little, quick, running step you'd take when you tried to cross the street against the light or catch a cab or look at a pretty woman? Remember how it felt to get out on a tennis court, all that spring in your legs? Remember the little bouncy hops, waiting for the opening kickoff when you played high school football? Anyway, try. Try to remember the *sense* of young movement.

Now for heaven's sake, don't start running for cabs or vaulting across police barricades. I don't want to be responsible for any fractures or coronaries. I just want you to reconstruct the *feeling*.

Now that you've got it, *walk!*

Walk at your usual tempo, but walk like the athlete you *were*. That's it, on the balls of your feet. Feet pointing straight ahead, as if you were wearing cleats. Lean forward a little, as if you were rushing at the net for a volley or following the football. Tummy in. Swing your arms free, fists half-clenched. Roll your shoulders, those enormous muscle-laden shoulders. Get your head up. Look at the far horizon where all adventures lie.

Now you're walking!

You're walking aggressively and athletically and youthfully, and *that's* the secret of John Wayne and all the others.

How have you been walking? You have shuffled and landed on the flat of your feet with your toes pointed out and your shoulders sagging. You've looked worn and hopeless and pitiable.

Now about sitting. Sit *up!* Cross your legs, if you will, but only if you have slim legs. Guys with scrawny polo-player legs look great with them elegantly crossed, but men with heavy thighs look like sacks of sod. What's more, they end up hiking the upper leg like grandma shuffling her corset. So, if your legs are heavier, cross them by putting your ankle over the knee, not the knee over the knee, savvy? Don't know what to do with your arms?

Cross them over your chest. Then square your shoulders. Main thing, if you sit upright, your belly will unfold.

What's the point of all this pulling and tugging?

To make you look younger, dummy! So many guys walk like old ladies and sit like frogs, and that includes guys who are only in their early thirties!

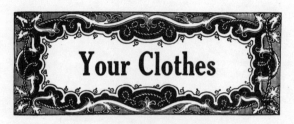

Your Clothes

**Looking Right While Still
Looking Like You**

Imitation

Look, even Rembrandt and Picasso were influenced by others. No shame in it. We all do (and should) snitch from those we admire.

In fashion there are, broadly speaking, two examples to follow:

(1) Socialites and rich people (they're really one and the same). Let's call 'em *poshrich*.

(2) Showbiz people and professional athletes. Let's call 'em *showjocks*.

Joe Namath, Sammy Davis, Jr., and Hugh Hefner are *showjock*.

Lord Louis Mountbatten and Gianni Agnelli are *poshrich*. The International Best-Dressed List is made up of the international *poshrich*.

These are the two main categories. Politicians are in the limelight too, of course, but they usually dress in democratic drab, so as not to offend a single voter. There are exceptions. Jimmy Walker was really *showjock* and Jack Kennedy *poshrich*.

But does everyone in a certain profession fall into one of the two categories? Uh-uh. It all depends on their ambition. For instance, Fred Astaire was a hoofer, and yet he's *poshrich*. Cary Grant began as a circus acrobat. He's *poshrich*.

Douglas Fairbanks, Jr. is *poshrich*. They are because they wanted to live in *poshrich* country.

Just the same, there's nothing wrong with being in *Showjock* country either. Any guy who gets his kicks out of the Namath style should imitate him. Half the young quarterbacks in football make like Namath. And *Playboy* has more readers than the Social Register. But it's mostly a young man's game. Usually people start out on the *showjock* route and work their way up toward imitating old money. Certainly the world's best resorts and biggest cities follow the *poshrich* road.

I'm not going to point in either direction. Sometimes the *poshrich* look silly and stuffy. More often, those who haven't Joe Namath's youth or build or Sammy Davis' flair look ridiculous trying to prance through Boutiqueland.

It's up to you which way you want to go.

Want to make it in the International-Jet-Set-Palm-Beach League? Try *poshrich*.

Want to make it in the Vegas–Hollywood–Third Avenue crowd? Try *showjock*.

Here's your reference material:

Showjock sources: television talk shows, the tabloid press, *Playboy*, *Penthouse*.

Poshrich: *Vogue* ('Goes to a Party'), *Town and Country*, *Palm Beach Pictorial*.

There are a few minor categories, but they shouldn't concern you. The music (pop) crowd. Too young for you, sorry. The Young-British-Lord, long-haired, velvet-suit-and-lace-ruffle division. Too young (and too lazy) for you, sorry. The guru and/or yippie-hippie-Commune set. Too young (and too kooky) for you, sorry.

By the way, there's one guy who can make it in *poshrich* country looking like Joe Namath.

You know who?

Joe Namath.

Starmaking

Having style . . . you wish you had the knack.
Well here's how.

It has to do with *starmaking*.

You have to be the starmaker.

You have to see your whole body as a performance. And, each day, you have to appoint the star
of that performance.

Sometimes it will be your *face*.

Suppose you've just come back from two
weeks in Jamaica and you're all crispy and sparkly
and healthy as well, and the martinis don't show.
Then the smart thing to do is to let your *face* star.

*Under*do everything else about you. Wear a

quiet shirt,
quiet tie,
quiet suit,
even quiet socks.

The focus *has* to be on your face. And it will
work. She'll say, "James, you look simply *marvelous*! Lost weight, too, didn't you?"

Don't distract from that expensive tan until it
has faded and the old oh-lord-I-could-use-some-
sleep or the oh-lord-did-I-hang-one-on look is back
on your puss. Then appoint something else to rule

for the day. Let's say, for example, your *shirt*.
Wear a

> wild striped shirt,
> solid color tie,
> solid color suit or blazer,
> plain socks,
> quiet shoes.

Everyone will say, "*Great* shirt, Oliver!"

But it can't be the shirt every day. Anything
done daily—well, almost anything—becomes a
bore. So make your suit the star, or a jacket, or
even your *tie*. Wear a

> yellow on red polka dot tie,
> cream colored shirt (plain),
> tan suit (plain),
> tan socks,
> brown loafer-type shoes.

The crowd will yell, "*Smashing* tie, Wood-
row!"

Get the idea?

You can let the *shoes* star, the kind with all
the gold gewgaws on them, and maybe the kind
made of crinkly patent leather. Or even, on certain
rambunctious days, just the *socks*, like those loud
red and blue checkered ones or the Argyles in
shades of yellow.

But don't do more than one loud thing at a
time. Don't expect people to applaud more than
one star at a time. More than one will turn them
off.

And be fickle. Be arbitrary. Go ahead and let
the morning mood guide you. Stand in front of
your closet and make everything in there tremble.
Tell every single item to measure up or it's off to

the thrift shop. Then point at your choice after keeping shoes, ties, socks, and suits in abject suspense.

I understand that one guy who pulls this stunt has a bright red tie which collapses in tears of gratitude each time he picks it. Another fellow has a tartan jacket which pleads and grovels until he wears it.

But remember, only one star at a time, or else you'll throw people into—thank you, Alvin Toffler —culture shock.

PS: Sometimes you can even let things *audition*. Like one shirt of mine which I have put through the wringer for three weeks and which is just too wild to wear. Maybe, one day, I'll introduce it to the world. But not yet. The world isn't ready.

The Necessities

There are some things you just can't do without. Richard III found out at Bosworth Field. Achilles found out after he bought those backless sandals. Abdul, the Eunuch, found out when he tried to make out with the Sultan's favorite wife. Yes indeed, there are some things you just can't do without!

Like the following:

A blazer. Preferably navy *mit* gold buttons. These days the double-breasted is fading again and the single-breasted is making its comeback. Whichever, if you don't have a blazer, get one. It can bridge almost all gaps. You can wear it for travel, for an informal evening, for *most* business occasions. (There are a few exceptions: very formal occasions, meetings with brand new clients, or when, for example, the chairman has made a big stink about not dressing too informally; or when you're just plain chicken.)

A navy suit. Preferably single-breasted. Preferably lightweight; you can wear lightweight suits summer and winter (since it rarely snows indoors). Single-breasted, because it's easier to sit in and that's what we do, mostly, sit.

A lightweight, tweed suit. Always single-breasted. Double-breasted tweed suits were only worn by grade B detectives in grade B movies in the grade B Thirties. Your tweed can be checked or Donegal or herringbone. Any way it's a "breakaway" suit, because you can take it apart and wear the jacket as a country jacket and the pants as a with-a-sweater separate.

A poplin suit. Maybe even the new stretchy kind (texturized, they call 'em, son), in tan. Again, single-breasted, and again, you can wear the pants as extras.

A featherweight, plain, medium gray suit. (Preferably S.B., natch.) It can serve for a semiformal evening, for formal business, or for good-looking travel, and the trousers can be etc., etc.

A knit suit. For travel. Try to get one *without* all the flaps on the pockets, the silly belt in the back, and the 1930s bi-swing back. Just a sleek, plain knit suit, in a neutral color like navy or gray or tan. You *must* have one for travel, because you can get on a plane, fly two hours, or five, get off, have a meeting, dine at your host's house, and still look quite respectable. At least the suit will look respectable. You may not. Your eyes will show bags before the suit does. Also, you don't have to holler for the valet if you're a lousy packer. Most knit suits forgive and forget. They're chums. Of course, they have drawbacks, as of this writing. They're a bit heavy and soggy. But it's worth it to know that your back won't wrinkle to the point where it looks like rhino hide.

And. You also need medium-gray slacks (two) and a pair of cavalry twill slacks (tan). Add some knit slacks (two), preferably plain-colored (gray and tan).

Above are the *musts.*

Armed thusly, you can make your appearance from Hong Kong to Rome, from La Jolla to Grosse Point, even if the rest of your wardrobe has been destroyed in a Kagoshima slide.*

Of course, you also need shirts, ties, shoes, raincoats, socks, evening wear and all that. But the above is the *big* stuff, the *institutional* stuff, the foundation from which all wardrobe wizardry stems.

---

* In truth, I don't expect you to be caught in one, unless you've got a hot business prospect on the island of Kyushu. In that case you're probably a Kagoshima resident and can go home and slip into your yukata, which is a sort of kimono. . . Oh, the heck with it. I'll tell you all about it in the Japan chapter. Relax.

Fit

There's an interplanetary distance between what most menswear stores describe as "good fit" and the real thing. Actually, clothes which truly fit seem to belong to a man's body, seem to *work* for him. For instance, you can tell Cary Grant's clothes and Fred Astaire's clothes *fit* because as these two men *move*—and both men move beautifully—clothes seem to be part of their bodies. On the other hand, Jimmy Stewart, who has never been known as a great fashion plate and who slouches and slumps, also has clothes which fit. They simply fit *him*. They do the trick. They are his partners. And thereby hangs the trick of fit. Clothes which fit must fit *you*, your body, your stance, your gait—your *physical personality*.

The moment of truth is when you have chosen the suit you want to buy, and they have summoned the man with the pins and the tape measure. It's now you and the suit, like two fighters right after the opening bell, or the matador watching his bull charge into the arena. For it is a contest. And remember that eventually *you must win*. The suit must submit. You *will* be boss . . . tell yourself that.

Your first round will be with the suit's sponsors: the salesman and the fitter. It is their function —no, their *duty*—to bully you. While the salesman stands by impatiently, pad and pencil in hand, the fitter will begin by telling you to stand up *straight*. Aha! That is your cue. Put your foot down, right there and then. Stand the way you always stand and tell them this is it, boys. Either fit me the way I always stand or forget the whole thing. They will mumble but submit. They will see the steel in your eyes, and obey.

Tell them to fit the pants first, *without* the jacket. Be sure they tighten the back with pins. Then sit down (carefully, mind you), to find out how it feels. Then, standing again, insist that the fronts of your trousers touch your shoes and that the backs are about ¾″ longer.

Next, get back into your old trousers* and have them fit the new suit jacket. Button it and stand relaxed, not bolt upright. See that the bottoms of the jacket sleeves are shortened to within 5½″ from the tips of your thumbs. (I personally prefer sleeves shortened to a 6″ setback, because I like to show a lot of shirt cuff. But I admit that's rather flashy.) Then move around in the jacket, see if it feels good. Stick your wallet into the pocket where you always carry it. In effect, give the jacket a test drive. Remember that you have a 98.6° pressing machine called your body which will steam the darn thing into place within a few weeks. And don't let them hand you any of that routine about "Your left shoulder is much lower than your right shoul-

---

* The new ones may be all bunched in back with pins.

der," tsk, tsk, shaken head, as though you were a
Frankenstein baby which they, poor souls, must
struggle to clothe. *No one is built symmetrically.*
But it doesn't matter a hoot, because no one ever
stands or sits bolt upright and squared away. Most
right-handed people have longer right arms and
legs; the opposite is true for the southpaw. You
are not a freak, I promise you.

Make a deal with the store to bring back the
suit in about a month so that they can make
adjustments after your body has made its own.
The sleeves may be too short or too long by then.
(Heavy fabrics like corduroy shrink slightly due to
wrinkling. Knits stretch back to their original, pre-
surgical state.)

When the suit arrives, take it out of the box
and wear it soon. Form it into shape. Break it to
your will. Bully it into submission. (Fred Astaire
once said he usually throws new suits against the
wall a few times until they know who's boss.)

That 5½″ gap between suit sleeve and thumb
tip will mean that about ½″ of shirt cuff will be on
display. (You really should not wear short sleeves
under a business suit.) Shirt cuffs should about hit
your wrist bone (almost covering your wristwatch). If you have to shove your shirt cuff way up
to read your watch, there's something wrong. And
if you have to hike up your suit sleeve to see your
shirt cuff, there's definitely something wrong.

The jacket waist should be *above* your real
waist (just below the bottom of your rib cage).
It's the most flattering place for a suit jacket to be
nipped in, and it's where the "waist" button of
your jacket should be. Same for double-breasted
jackets. By raising the waist, you look taller and

your legs look longer and, *in toto*, you look super, Osbert.

Anyway. Don't let 'em push you around. Not the suit. Not the salesman. Not the fitter. Listen to Toto. He knows.

The Jocks

Sorry. This chapter is not about an athlete's invisible means of support. Rather, this is a friendly chat with those of my contemporaries who are superjocks, athletes, body builders, and/or Atlas devotees.

You found out long ago that with that 18″ neck, the 48″ chest, the huge biceps, and the 33″ waist there is *nothing* you can buy to fit. Nothing!

Every pair of pants has to be recut when you buy a suit so the back pockets meet at the center.

Shirts to fit your neck? Hah! Try and find them.

The only outfit you look great in is a swimsuit.

But suppose you who *are* a jock, a football player, and basketball player who's been at it since high school and who may now even make your living at it? My first advice is, great chunky bodies are never ideal for elegant clothes. For one thing, your legs are heavy and slim pants make you look like you're standing on liverwursts.

Don't try to look too "in." Most avant-garde clothing is built for scrawny kids. Besides, you're an overwhelming-looking guy, a big guy, an impressive guy. Don't gild the lily by wearing super hip clothes.

You don't know it, but the rest of us, the men who aren't professional athletes, laugh at athletes who overdo the fashion *shtick*.

And eventually you will stop being a pro athlete. You'll look for managerial work, probably *outside* of sports. You can't afford to be thought of as a self-indulgent muscle freak. You'll need to be taken seriously.

Look at Frank Gifford and Kyle Rote. They always manage to stay . . . businesslike.

By the time you're fifty, people won't remember your heroic deeds. They'll only see what's in front of their noses.

Now that I've chewed you out, here comes the advice. Go to those big-man and tall-man shops, but beware: dodge *their* idea of fashionable gear. Hunt up and down the aisles until you find something *quiet and conservative*.

I said it before and I'll say it again: Don't over-overwhelm people. Underwhelm them!

Pockets

Chum, you're carrying too much junk in your pockets. Yes, you are! No matter what you tell me. I know it; it's too much.

Okay, you need your credit cards. But how many? Diner's Club and American Express and Master Charge and BankAmericard and Mobil and Texaco and Shell and Gulf and Getty and Air Travel Card and store cards and The Great Computer knows what else.

Well, that's a lot of bunk. You'll find that most of the time you duplicate cards. For instance, it should be *either* Express or Diner's. Most places accept both. And the oil cards? Most dealers, too, take Diner's or Express. You don't need most store cards. If you have an account, they'll check on it and use your driver's license as identification.

Most of the credit-card cases with the fold-out "snake" are fat and unnecessary. Consolidate your cards and then use one of those slim little cases you get for business cards. That's all. You can slide it into the breast pocket of your shirt. No bulge. Honest. No bilge.

What else do you carry?

A secretary-type note pad? Thick. Bulky. Instead, have your wife, your secretary, or your gal (maybe they overlap) cut you some plain 3″ by 4″ cards and stick them into your outside jacket pocket. You can write a ton of notes, using both sides—just write small. Yes, of course, you'll carry a pen. That's no big deal. What else?

Cigarettes? Well, that one I can't lick. Keys? Best to carry them on a ring or chain, not in a case. They're harder to lose when they clank. Money? Folded in a back pocket, buttoned if possible, or in a clip in your forward pants pocket, but *not* in one of those fat wallets, ham-hock style.

In fact, here's my suggestion. When you're in your hometown, carry money and one credit card like the Express or Master Charge, and that's all. And the little note cards and your pen. You can leave all the other cards at home. Of course you must carry your driver's license, but that can fit into that flat little business-card case I spoke of before, along with three of your calling cards. Chances are you have charge accounts all over your hometown anyway.

For traveling in the U.S., add a *few* cards (airlines, airline clubs, one oil company).

For travel abroad, your passport. Being a big, fat, lumbering thing, you're best off carrying it in your hand luggage. You could also carry a flat 10″ by 12″ zipper case—to hold your passport, a paperback book for the plane, some maps and brochures as well as any business papers you need. Most of the time you can leave your passport in your hotel. It's safe there (at the desk), and nobody asks you for it except to exchange money, which you can do at the hotel or at airports where you've got your passport in your hand luggage. Get it?

Glasses. Ah yes, glasses. If you need them just for reading, get the "grandpa" kind, the half-moon ones. They're slim and fit into your breast pocket.

Anyway, some of the things I said will drive you up the wall. You'll be furious. You'll tell me you can't live without your telephone directory, or customers card file, which is one-foot thick, or, for all I know, your Amateur Morse Code Operator's Certificate.*

But if I've made you think a bit, if I've provoked you into spinning off (how's that for executive talk?) some of your excess junk, I'm proud of myself. I've debulged your pockets. I've struck again!

---

* A guy I know has his fifty most important phone numbers (legal and otherwise) typed on a small card the size of a business card. Try it. It works. And you can swallow it in case of emergency. Have you ever tried to chew a little black book?

The Fancy Belt

Fancy, wide belts are great ... *IF*.

The condition? That you are a young kid with slim hips. Any wide belt (2" and up) *above size 36* (meaning you have a real 36" waist, not that you're squeezing your 38" pot into a 36" belt) is absolutely no good. Its extra width only makes you look extra fat. It emphasizes your midship beam. Fat belts are only for those who can circle slim middles.

And even if your waist qualifies but your bottom is too big, it's no go. The rear view of big belt and big can is a big horror.

But you can hide any roll *above* the belt. (It's got to go *somewhere*, doesn't it?) Only don't wear a rib-hugging sweater or shirt. Wear a loose sweater or shirt. That way it will look as if those cloth folds above the belt are the sweater or shirt. Nobody will guess that they are filled with your spare tire.

Dig, Daddy?

Shirt Tales

To begin with, the shirt is probably the most modern piece of men's apparel that we wear. To many men in many businesses, it is the main form of fashion expression.

Why the shirt? Why not the suit jacket, the sport coat, the sweater?

Because 80 percent of today's business blokes —from shipping foreman to executive vice-president—work in their shirt-sleeves.

Because nine-tenths of our days are spent sitting at desks in offices and we might as well be bare-assed below table level.

There are already many industries where business suits are not required. If you're in the oil business and you zoom from well to well by helicopter, who needs a pin stripe? If you're a small-plane dealer in Florida, do you need your executive duds? If you're in the construction business in New Mexico, do you need your office armor? The heck you do. Unless you're going to meet the bankers. Many business clubs and restaurants in America (in the *real* America, not Madison Avenue or Beverly Hills) allow you to lunch in your shirt-sleeves. Now I'm not ringing the death knell for the jacket, but the fact is most of us dump it as soon as we get to our desk.

What's more, we now have red shirts and pink shirts and striped shirts and multistriped shirts and polka dot shirts and geometric-print shirts and knit shirts. That already allows a guy a lot of freedom of expression.

The Europeans? They're just beginning to get wise to the modern way of life. Ten years ago no European could understand why I always had pockets on my shirts. Today they know: they work in their shirtsleeves just like us, and they need some place to stash their pens.

Lastly, in our air-conditioned and centrally heated lives, we certainly don't need our jackets for *warmth*. Indoor climate variations are disappearing, and ours is an indoor life. Even a car is indoors. So is a plane.

Half the guys I know walk from house into garage into car into parking ramp into office into business luncheon, and reverse the whole process at night without ever leaving a temperate 70°, even if it's ten below or one hundred above outside.

A guy I know traveled from Los Angeles over the North Pole to Helsinki without ever putting on his overcoat. In our fathers' days that would have sounded like a Jules Verne adventure, but you can do the same. Just call S.A.S. and tell them to charge it.

Even more interesting: No one tsk-tsked my friend. Everyone is used to the idea of a guy sitting on a plane in his shirtsleeves. Okay, okay, so we're witnessing the corruption of manners, the collapse of Western civilization, and what is the world coming to and so on. Fact is, more and more, the shirt is becoming the outer shell of a man. The suit jacket still has an important role and will have for many years to come, but it has become the *outer* jacket and has placed the overcoat on the endangered species list.

The reason for this preamble is to point out how important shirts are and will be.

Let's have a go at the business shirt first. Here are the general categories: Long-sleeved and short-sleeved, plain collars and button-downs. (The tab collar and the eyelet-type collar-pin collar have bitten the dust for the time being. Though you can never be sure a collar style is defunct. Even the separate or stiff collar, bless it, the mastodon of collardom, occasionally surfaces among British bankers and French postal officials. But then, I assume there are very few of those among my readers.)

The shirt of the moment, the hero of the day, is the long-sleeved, pointed-collar, business shirt. In its most avant-garde form it has a two-button barrel cuff (as opposed to the French cuff which needs cuff links.) Collars are fairly long and, when worn by connoisseurs, are flared slightly. This flare stuff is not a prerogative of aristocratic birth. You, the wearer, make the collars flare simply by sticking your thumb and forefinger under the things and rolling them upward. If they have stays, just bend the little devils. The reason for the flare is that your collar doesn't look so stiff and new. (As you will discover over and over, clothes should look as if you've had them for a while, not store-fresh. Casually rich, you know. A smidgen of affectation. But you're allowed, okay?)

One advantage of the self-button cuff is that you can't lose or forget your cuff links; you won't end up cursing yourself one morning in the Dallas Hilton as you search under the chest of drawers for the pair that got away and your French cuffs flap around like elephants' ears. The other advantage is that if you point at some impressive curve on the sales graph, your French cuff won't get stuck on the outside of your suit jacket sleeve. Unless you happen to have custom-made shirts with very tight French cuffs. But they cost a lot of money and the laundry treats custom jobs like any other vulgar shirt. Rip. Tear. Shred.

Not that I have anything against French-cuffed shirts. They look great with very dressy suits, like charcoal pin-stripeds or navy double-breasteds. But too often the French cuff is an excuse to show off the sort of cuff links most hookers would be ashamed to wear as earrings. You know, the huge, jeweled and enameled and Florentined kind of atrocities. Those are no-nos. Please don't fall for any talk of their superb design and craftsmanship. They're vulgar. Period. Like brocade tuxedos or stiletto-toed shoes or jade-green suits. If you wear cuff links, make them rather small and neat. *Please*!

About the button-down collar. Until a few years ago it was the mark of success. Wall Street, Ivy League, University Club, private yacht, you name it. Then they became too popular to stay prestigious, and, darn it, they slipped from favor. Which is a shame, really, because they are very contemporary and soft and casual and right, and most men look good in them. Mind you, there are certain old-line socialites who have always worn them and will always wear them, because these fellows are above the storms of fashion. But most of us will have to wait a while for their return. And return they will, this I promise you. So meantime, if you own them, don't give them up for adoption.

The short-sleeved business shirt. Yes, the short-sleeved business shirt. It's wrong, cornball, slobovian. And yet, in many cases it's right. It's right when you spend 95 percent of your time in your shirtsleeves and you're working in an informal town with a warm climate, like San Diego, say. And it's right where the custom among executives is to wear short-sleeved shirts—like, well, like San Diego. For the occasional jacket wearer in an informal town . . . okay, short sleeves. Like in San Diego. Or did I mention that?

But if you're traveling to New York, don't. No use giving an impression which you'll have to be brilliant to overcome. ("He looks like a hick, but he's really brilliant.") Nobody should ever have to be brilliant anyway. It's too tiring.

And now, the gut question. White or colorful? Solid or striped or checked or print? Well, let's reach back to the beginning of this section. Most of the time you are seen in your shirt. What impression do you want to make? Are you forever glued to the I'm-an-executive-and-proud-of-my-superior-position image? Do you think that any shirt other than a white shirt is frivolous, flamboyant and unreliable? Frankly, if you do, you're not just stuffy—you're naive. The colored business shirt was *invented* by the old Groton-Princeton-Newport crowd. Brooks Brothers was selling them blue and pink and yellow when the rest of the world was smugly secure in respectable white shirts. Because the old Ivy League boys felt above that sort of thing.

And here's another point: In the days when executives were stuck in their hometown, the white shirt would do. But today there are many of us who breakfast at home, go through an afternoon of conferences and then have a business dinner, without a chance to change. After that sort of abuse, a blue shirt looks a lot neater. There is nothing sadder than a white shirt that has lost its virginity.

About stripes, checks, prints: once you've broken the white-shirt shackles, have a fling. All the compliments you'll receive will reassure you, this I guarantee. But one warning. Be careful about wearing patterned shirts with patterned ties. It's tricky business. Usually there can only be one star to an outfit. If it's the shirt, so be it. If it's the tie, so be it. But two stars around the same throat . . . well, they are bound to try to upstage one another.

(I have a simple rule for myself: I never wear a patterned tie with a patterned shirt. And I always wear a patterned tie with a plain shirt. Unless I wear crazy socks. Then I wear a plain tie with a plain shirt and crazy socks. Unless I wear a crazy suit. Then I wear every dingle-dangle thing plain, except the suit. See the chapter entitled *Star-making*.)

How should a shirt fit? A business shirt should have about four inches of play around the waistline, not much more. Most stock shirts are carefully computered for the average waist. If you don't fit a "big-brand" shirt, cut out the booze, Bernard. The cuff should end near the bottom of your wrist bone, just above your wristwatch, or maybe covering it halfway (unless it's a short-sleeved shirt, in which case that would be one helluva trick!).

Sport shirts are much simpler. Knit shirts are the most flattering, but they're sometimes warm. If your heart yearns for wild prints, go, baby! Remember that it's easy to cheat away the spare roll if you wear your sport shirt *outside* the pants.

Want to know the really razzle-dazzle, super chic way to wear a sport shirt? Cuffs rolled up to just below the elbow, collar *up* and the four top buttons (make that five top buttons) unbuttoned. Provided you have a tanned chest and at least a semblance of a Burt Lancaster physique. Then you can also wear a St. Christopher medal or a silver dollar or a Monte Carlo chip on a gold chain, bouncing around on that sun-tanned chest. Style and flair. Try it. You'll slaughter 'em, Eric!

On Your Toes

All I'm going to ask is that you use your head when you consider your feet. No need to lug around extra pounds à *pied*. No need to struggle with shoelaces in the Seventies.

Nearly all American executives in their late thirties or above (anyone here above?) has at one time or other been in love with the WASP–Oxford–blood-red cordovan, the one with the thick soles. It came out of the era of imitating the Ivy-League–Wall-Street boys who wore these ugly boats on their feet because cordovans were one of the clenched-jaw, social-register symbols. Doesn't make sense to me; never did. We spend 90 percent of our life sitting on our duffs in offices, cars, planes. Why should a modern city man wear heavy-soled outdoor "mudders"? In summer they're too hot. In winter you have to wear galoshes or overboots anyway. So why not wear lightweight, soft-soled shoes? Bad for your feet? The heck they are. The Indians wore featherweight deerskin moccasins, and did you ever hear of an Indian with fallen arches? If you *walk* right, feet pointing straight ahead, using the balls of your feet for spring, you won't need arch support.

About laces: Anyone who has ever groaned

over a broken shoelace, knotted it and then had it hurt him all day will know what I mean. After all, we here in America pioneered the modern-day loafer-moccasin long before the Italians ever heard of the ones with the metal trim. So pamper yourself; wear slip-ons. With all sorts of buckles and ornaments. Go ahead.

About boots: They're okay when they're lightweight and short and worn on a sloppy day. But the knee-high kind is kid stuff, latter-day storm trooper. As for stuffing your pants into them—silliest thing I ever heard, unless you're living in North Dakota and walking to the barn in winter. But on a city street? Come off it. What's more, your pants will look like hell.

Patent leather mocs are now okay for daytime wear, not just for spruced-up evenings. If they're sort of low and light, they look rather nice. In fact, they can take the place of highly shined street shoes. I like the black ones best. Sometimes, for tan or brown suits, I like dark brown. I'd skip the blue, green, orange, or bright-yellow sort. They look too Russian Ballet.

Now about those high heels and/or platform soles they sell in so-called fashion shoe boutiques: Most guys in high heels teeter around like 1950 high-school girls on their way to the junior prom. It's a fast-moving world, Erskine. Don't hamper yourself. Even rodeo cowboys have given up their high heels.

If you wear high heels to make yourself feel taller, forget it. (Unless you make love with your boots on.)

Hats

In one way hats have had it. In another way, they're only just coming back to life.

The old "You're not an executive unless you wear a hat on the 8:40" business is kaput. The Madison-Avenue-helmet syndrome is over. In the cities you rarely see business hats, and, except for hatcheck girls, no one is shedding any tears. It was idiotic to buy your hat back a quarter at a time from every restaurant, club, bar, and hotel in the country.

But the hat for leisure and sports is just beginning. Tennis hats and boating hats and beach hats and golf hats and let's-get-loaded-because-we're-in-Bermuda-whoopee! hats are being snapped up because they're great fun. They allow you to masquerade as your innermost favorite hero. Elephant hunter? Go! America's Cup sailor? Go! Rod Laver? Go!

Only thing is to keep the masquerade in its place. No room for Caribbean pirates on State Street. No need for cowboys—midnight, drugstore, or Texan—on Fifth Avenue.

There are really only two reasons left for the old city chapeaux: rain and cold. Some anti-umbrella men like a roll-up rain hat, particularly when traveling. You can stow the thing in a raincoat pocket. And some men like the furry Cossack-style hat for freezing days. Fine, though I've wondered why no one turns the flaps down, as ear warmers. If you're going to wear the things, it seems silly not to let them do their stuff.

One interesting phenomenon: Men who discarded business hats for work and who enthusiastically adopted sports hats on weekends and vacations have been donning leisure-type hats for city wear as well. In fact, there might be a big return of the Tyrolean-type sports hat, the loden-green ones in velour or rough felt, for the city. In case I could turn out to be wrong, I hereby urge you to consider Tyrolean-type hats for fall and winter city wear. That way I'll turn out to be right. Maybe.

Under the Outside Man

Let's discuss what salesladies in department stores once called "intimate apparel" (meaning that you must get intimate with them to buy the apparel, they hope).

In short, underwear.

A recent survey revealed that most modern men prefer knit Jockey shorts to the boxer type. Don't ask us how the informal survey was taken. The women researchers involved are very stiff-necked about that sort of thing. *Very* stiff-necked.

It's a fact. The so-called boxer short (of course no boxer in his right mind would wear boxer shorts under his trunks) seems to be *through*. It probably *has* to do with the heavier layer of cloth which you have to fold underneath the new tight-fitting pants.

It's *Jockey*-type shorts, friends; those tight, knitted little devils which can go all the way down to almost-bikinis, which give you moral and physical support, and which leave no telltale folds under your tight-assed pants.

They're the winners in today's underworld.

Now about the undershirt.

Really needed?

No.

There's a whole contingent of guys who insist
that they *must* wear an undershirt, else it gets to
be messy time in midsummer. Maybe they're right.
Personally, I don't think so. But if it makes them
feel more secure, what the heck.

But here's the best part: They now make underwear in the wildest, the craziest, the darndest
colors and prints, and you really owe it to yourself
to give vent to your sense of subsurface adventure.
Think of it: You're at a business meeting, dressed
in subdued gray, saying subdued gray things to a
subdued gray business prospect. . . But wait; your
heart is aflutter because under all that gray is a
pair of yellow shorts with red polka dots and he
can't see them. Makes a grown man get all tearful.
Deep down inside.

The Locker Room

The locker room is a dead giveaway. Guys come in dressed to the teeth: pressed, styled, shined, and sprayed. Then they get into their gym outfits. The crummiest, cruddiest, rankest, rattiest gym outfits north of Tijuana.

One jockstrap? *For six months*? Come on, now! One T-shirt now and forever? A lifelong pair of tennis shorts? We're not even mentioning sweat socks. They're named to perfection.

These same guys make a big fashion to-do about their tennis and golf togs because they're on public display. But when it comes to the privacy of a gym . . . who cares? Well, I damn well care. May I remind you that we've all got noses and eyes, even if we're your middle-aged locker neighbors and not the pretty girls on the tennis courts or golf greens.

Mister, have a heart!

Around the Water

Most of us pass thirty-five, eventually. As a penalty for having made it, we have to rethink our appearance. We just ain't as pretty as we were at twenty-five. Sorry. That's the way the belly bounces.

Even the super athletes and those who keep telling us that they "can eat anything and never put on weight" develop a case of the *dangles*. The *dangles* have nothing to do with sexual prowess. They simply refer to the little rolls which gather at the lower part of the back when our formidable back muscles follow Newton's Law and settle downward.

Secondly, we get the *puckers*. They describe the results when a muscle, mostly in the chest region, just isn't as firm as when you rowed for Yale.

Lastly, we get a bit more hairy . . . and sometimes *gray*-hairy.

All of this doesn't matter a damn in the boardroom or in the bedroom. In the words of the song: When somebody loves you, it's no good unless they love you, *all the way*. After all, some of the world's great lovers look like Onassis in their swimsuits. In fact, Onassis looks like Onassis in his swimsuit.

But face facts: not all the world loves a lover and many strangers who stand in awe of you when you're in your clothes merely say "Aw . . ." when they look at you in a swimsuit.

And I'm not even speaking about the unspeakables, like varicose veins and scars from kidney operations. I'm just mentioning the usual, normal devastation of Old Pop Time.

Don't let all of this depress you. The only thing which really hurts is the collapse of self-delusion, and I know that all of the things I said above are already clear to you. You didn't need *me* to tell you what the years have wrought, right?

Now, a few ways of cheating the public, a few bits of razzle-dazzle.

Most men's legs are okay to the age of seventy. But if you really have lousy-looking legs, the answer is to wear long cotton pants. Wear them without socks and shoes, à la "beachcomber." The effect can be very snazzy and devil-may-care.

About the *dangles* and the *puckers*. Wear *loose* overshirts or beach tops or beach parkas or sweaters—over a bare chest—and don't take them off until the second you're going in the water. In fact, wear them to the *edge* of the water and then strip, bending forward to pull up the back muscles. Leave them within easy reach (the clothes, not the muscles) so you can re-dress seconds after you emerge from the briny. If you're afraid of getting the shirt or jacket wet, bring a towel, use it fast and then back into your covering. Again, leave the front unbuttoned. Most men's chests look okay. It's the side silhouette which shows you can indeed remember Pearl Harbor.

About the suntan you won't get because you're wearing long pants and/or a beach top:

don't worry. No one ever sees you bare-chested at the bank or your broker's. All they see is your face and your hands. I find the allover suntan highly overrated—except for nudists.

About lovers: No one makes love in a bright, spotlit room. The ideal light is somewhat hazy; so who the heck can tell about your tan? Even then, you can play the game by using your robe or (if it's in *her* palazzo) a towel or two until the moment of truth.

Now to review: Cover the dangers (back, side silhouette, bad legs), and expose the good parts (face, arms, hand, chest, ankles, feet).

If you have to be bare, make it fast.

Finally, knit swimsuits and elastic swimsuits tend to accentuate the dangles. Try canvas-type or sailcloth-type shorts which really look like walk shorts or cut-off jeans. And, for an extra measure of caution, buy them a size too large.

Black Tie

On charity invitations they say "Black Tie." Among the jet set they say, "We're dressing" (meaning, I suppose, that anything but black tie is bare-assed). The more plebeian speak of "going formal" or "wearing a tuxedo." Among waiters and musicians it's still just a "tux."

It all adds up to the same thing: wearing your monkey suit.

The average business guy only has to worry about dress formalities at business conventions and charity balls. And once in a while at the country club. Like New Year's Eve. Or maybe for a wedding and carryings-on of that sort. The jet setter has only to worry about it in New York and Palm Beach, because in London, Rome, and Paris they don't bother too often these days.

Until a few years ago, many people rented their dinner clothes and I suppose it was okay; I have nothing against rental clothes (like who the hell owns a cutaway for weddings?). But all in all, I think it's a good investment to own your own dinner suit or tuxedo or whatever you want to call it. Avoid the faddish and it will serve you for a long time. It's just, well, *nicer* to wear your own clothes.

Now, there's an odd split that takes place at different social levels. Surpisingly, it is the hard hats who wear fancy-shmantzy tuxedos with super frilly shirts, sometimes in pink or blue with all kinds of pansy ruffles. Whereas the supposedly sissified upper "clawsses," the international jet-set crowd, wear very, very quiet dinner suits with very plain white shirts. You'll never see an international society feller with an eight-button maroon Edwardian tuxedo and rose-red ruffled shirt trimmed in pink lacing with a maroon satin bow tie.

Never.

Never, never, never.

On the other hand, great, big, hulking football tackles somehow decide to wear all the gook.

Once in a blue moon you'll see a jet-set type with a black velvet suit, but it'll be cut very simply (single-breasted, one-button) and will be worn with a plain white shirt and black bow tie.

Maybe, because the jet-set fellers spend so much time in their dinner suits, they treat them as normal gear; maybe they think it's not complimentary to a woman to out-ruffle and out-puce her. Be that as it may, the "chic" man wears a *very simple* tuxedo, while the plumbing salesman at his annual wing-ding pretends he's Errol Flynn.

I have spelled out all the above because I want *you* to make up your mind which it's to be: simple or fancy. I suppose if it's a once-a-year whoop-it-up of the Grand Order of Swamp Buffalo, and you want to look as you'd never dare to look when sober, well, then, go ahead. But I must confess that the average business Joe looks like a jackass in emerald brocade or in a mauve ruffled shirt. Sorry. The credibility gap between his normal life and his formal clothes is too wide. Instead of

feeling and looking "formal," he looks "costume party" and probably acts it to boot. In a way it's the same old lampshade-on-the-head gag.

My personal preference? I'll confess. While I'm all for color and flair and flash in my daytime clothes, I like my evening suits simple and black. Single-breasted, with a plain white shirt (no frills or ruffles) and a simple black bow tie. I even have little plastic "gold" buttons sewn onto a normal button-cuff white shirt. They just stay attached and go through the laundry. I don't have to fiddle with those devilish little studs and slippery cuff links when I dress up. My tuxedo must be feather-weight (I dance; don't you?), and that makes it easy to pack, too.

Do I tie my own bow tie? Another confession: no. You can get very good ready-made ones. I'd suggest the butterfly kind, not the niggling little triangles or those sad flaps you tuck under your collar. They're too Las Vegas.

If you don't believe me, get a hold of your wife's *Town and Country* and look at the party photographs. If you can show me a man in super fancy gear at a really "social" party, I'll eat my bow tie, which happens to be made of satin.

Weddings and Funerals

There are two time-honored rituals which are under attack. Weddings and funerals. Marriage may disappear one of these days. Death, no doubt, will be around a little longer.

As for the services, it's also true that funerals will survive longer than weddings. No one has, as yet, devised a pop funeral.

It seems ridiculous to talk about how a guest should dress for these occasions, but you'd be surprised. Many men are too fashion-shaky to be sure. Here are some rules.

An old-fashioned wedding. This is the kind where there are rehearsals and rented cutaways and fathers of the bride moaning over bills and relieved mothers of the bride and ushers and bridesmaids and until-death-do-us-part oaths. You wear a white shirt and a dark suit, unless it's a summer garden wedding. In that case you can wear blazer and white slacks with shirt and tie.

All of the above applies only to guests. If you're part of the wedding—on the staff, so to speak—you get your orders from the boss, usually the best man. Talk him into the club jacket (normal, short, black, business-type jacket, not the

tailed-type cutaway) with striped pants and gray
vest. Most man can't handle tailed jackets. If you
have to wear cutaways, practice the old concert-
pianist-sitting-down-at-piano gesture. You reach
back and flip up the tails to the side. Admittedly
it's a ridiculous motion and can make you look like
a long-gowned dowager sitting down in her box at
the opera, but you must suffer to be smart.

Second, third, or fourth remarriage. This is
one of the type held at the penthouse of a friend
or in a small hotel with the children on both sides
there to watch. Wear a business suit and a white
shirt, even if you're a witness. No one in his right
mind goes through a formal, pristine, virginal wedding ceremony for a second or third time round.
If he tries, talk him out of it.

Funerals. Now they are another matter. They
deserve to be treated with a certain air of sadness,
even if the protagonist's departure has spread glee
deep in the hearts of the spectators. (As they said
of the deceased at one Hollywood tycoon's funeral
which was absolutely *swamped* with mourners:
"He was right! Give the people what they want to
see and they'll come in droves. . . .") Whatever
your inclinations, assume a posture of restrained
grief and wear a white shirt, business suit, and
plain tie, *preferably black*. If you don't want to
let go of your personality entirely, wear sunglasses
with your dark suit, white shirt, black tie. All the
Hollywood types do that. It supposedly hides the
tear-worn eyes and deep, sad pouches. Actually, it
hides the usual bloodshot eyes and booze-worn
pouches.

If you have a real whoopee luncheon on the
calendar shortly after the funeral, bring a kicky tie

and shirt in your briefcase and change after the interment.

If you're the (how can I put it?) central figure in a funeral, you don't have to worry about your wardrobe. Someone will lay it out for you, I'm sure.

The Hospital

Sorry, but eventually it seems to get around to all of us. Sometimes minor—"Just a few days, Mr. Harrison, and you'll be going home as good as new"—and sometimes major, which we won't think about now. Sometimes planned, sometimes . . . whammo. The hospital.

If the operation is long-anticipated, if you and the surgeon have a date of long standing (one always makes it far, far in advance, not from foresight but from fear), prepare as if you're going on a one- or two-week trip. Try as soon as possible to get out of those clinical-looking hospital gowns and wear your own pajamas and robe. Bring cologne. Bring a sun lamp. Bring note pads. Bring pens. (Don't bring books. People send 'em.) Turn the hospital room into *your* room.

It's not only good for *your* morale, it also helps your *visitors*, who are all too ready to tsk-tsk and write you off as a ruin.

Of course, if you get carted to the hospital for an emergency, you can't be expected to haul along a sauna bath. But as soon as the medicos stop looking anxious, get your wife or current girl friend to bring your own gear. You'd be surprised what a whiff of good aftershave can do for you and your visitors.

If your own pajamas, robe, and slippers are sort of tattered, this is a great time for getting new ones. Get someone to shop for you if you're flattened unexpectedly. Vanity in the hospital is not only *not* sinful, it's a *must*. Vain patients, my doctor-friends tell me, seem to recover more quickly.

Private Fashion Manners

What have you got against your wife and children? Nothing? Then why do you dress like that at home? Aren't they entitled to a pleasant view of you, Mortimer?

You get home each evening and take off your suit and roll yourself into a moth-eaten robe and a pair of scuffed slippers. Nice? Or it's Sunday and you turn up in a sad pair of worn-down corduroys and the golf shirt with the hole in the left armpit. Nice? The hell it is.

I'm not suggesting that you wear a blazer, white flannels, and an ascot to mow the lawn. But I do suggest that you wear nifty coveralls or some great knit pants with a knit shirt or crisp, clean Levi's with a handsome wide belt and a body-sweater (the last outfit only if your waist is okay).

Think of it this way. How would you dress if:

Your wife tells you that your nineteen-year-old daughter is coming home for the weekend with three of her long-legged college roommates?

Or a business associate will be dropping over with his wife, whom you've never met but who is much younger than her husband (she's his second) and who looks smashing in the photo on his desk?

Oh, so now you know what to wear around

the house that Sunday, do you? Now you get the idea!

Just don't overreact. As I said before, no white flannels. No ascot. No need to have your own family burst out laughing.

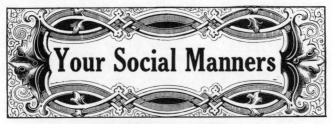

Your Social Manners

**A Few Thoughts
About Faring With *Savoir***

At Table

Okay, so you say I have my nerve.

Here you are a grown man and I'm talking to you about table manners, like you're a kid, for Chrissake.

All right, I've got my nerve.

But there are a helluva lot of successful men with great clothes and handsome mugs and everything going for them who *eat like day laborers*.

I don't expect you to eat European style, holding your fork in the left hand and your knife in the right. The American system is good enough, despite all the fork switching from left hand to right. But do, at least, hold your fork like a civilized adult. I've seen plenty of well-educated executives hold their forks in their clenched fists when they're cutting their meat, like Macbeth grabbing the fatal dagger. Please, hold your fork like a pencil and at the *end* of the handle, not clutched near the prongs. Then, when you're ready to switch, grab it the same way with your right hand.

Butter your roll on the butter plate, not in your hand. Don't blow on your soup. Stir it with your spoon, while the clouds rise. (As for restaurants, boiling hot soup and boiling hot coffee are the mark of the hash house.) Sit up and bring the food to your mouth. Don't hunch over the plate. Try not to talk with your mouth full, no matter how important the sales pitch. And when you're through leave your fork and knife lying next to each other on the plate, not spread-eagled.

When you go to a restaurant, don't stand at the entrance like a draftee waiting for his physical. Take a few steps inside. Then the maitre d' will come at you faster. Fix him with a strong gaze and give him your name: "I'm Mr. Dalrymple." As if he should know. Ten to one he'll say, "Ah yes, Mr. Dalrymple," and take you to your appointed table. Sounds silly, but more men walk into restaurants and get tongue-tied. "Er, I have a, well, reservation. For three. At one." Then you get the examination. "Your name, sir?" "Dalrymple." Then the maitre d' checks the list like an immigration agent looking for undesirables. Anyway, try the "I'm Mr. Dalrymple." Unless, of course, your name is Wellsby. In which case "Dalrymple" won't do you much good, even with a steady gaze.

If a restaurant where you've made a lunch reservation asks you to wait at the bar, wait at the bar that one time, but don't ever go back there. Any restaurant that takes a luncheon reservation knows that you're on a tight schedule. If they don't have your table ready, tough on them. Never tip a captain after he's kept you waiting for a reserved table.

Don't insist that everyone booze it up before lunch. More guys than ever are passing up their prelunch drinks and would be happier if you don't urge them. Whatever sales pitch you want to make won't sound any better because your guest has had one drink. And if he gets loaded, it won't matter what you said.

Unless you speak great French or Italian, don't try it with the captain. You'll make an ass of yourself with your table companions. You're in America. Speak American.

And don't chatter with the waiter. He's there to serve you, not to entertain you. In his eyes, you'll rate according to your tip, not your conversation.

If you're the host, and there are ladies present, take the whole order and give it to the captain. If it's men only, everyone is on his own. And remember *who* ordered *what*, so you can tell the waiter when he brings the hash.

In spite of all those magazine articles, you don't have to be a wine expert. Let the headwaiter or *sommelier* suggest. He won't steer you wrong. Don't make too much wine-tasting fuss. Just sip and say okay and don't pay too much attention. The chances of your getting bad wine are only one in five hundred.

Also remember that, generally speaking, first-rate restaurants have smallish portions. Cheap restaurants have big portions. In a luxury restaurant, if you want more, ask for it. They assume you're not starving and will serve you a civilized portion to begin with. The cheap restaurant tries to show you you're "getting value for your money." Also interesting—isn't it—good restaurants have waiters and cheap restaurants have waitresses. Don't know why. But that's the way it is.

If you have to explain something in writing to your companions, don't use the tablecloth. One of the waiters will give you a pad. Unless you're Raymond Loewy, or Dali. Then they'll auction off the tablecloth.

No matter how funny something is, or no

matter how important your guest is (so his joke seems funnier than it really is), don't go into hysterics in a restaurant. There's nothing as disturbing as the man who pounds the table and collapses in laughter, like a hyena while mating. (I understand that hyenas laugh during mating season, which I can't blame them for.)

If someone you don't recognize hails you from across the room, wave back and say, "How are you?" or "Nice to see you!" You'll never know whom you might have snubbed otherwise.

And if *anyone* stops at your table to speak to you, get to your chubby feet. If he's a "nobody," it'll make you look all the better.

If someone stops to gab and you don't remember his name, point at your table mate and say, "You remember Jack Hornspur, don't you?" Then the stranger will introduce himself. (Another ploy: If you're at a convention with your wife and you're worried about remembering names—even of clients who send in $50,000 orders—train your wife to put out her hand and introduce herself immediately, forcing the other party to say his own name.)

When the meal is over, look over your bill. That makes sense. But don't make it a corporate study. It embarrasses your guests.

Once you've signed the check, turn it face down for the waiter to collect. No one at your table need know what you've spent and what you've tipped.

If you pay cash (Holy Moses, *cash*?), tuck the dough under the check. Same as if you signed.

Why did I do this whole chapter?

Because it's getting to be a small world and you'll be hosting Europeans and Japanese and South Americans. And they'll think you're some kind of oaf unless you *eat* decently. And because many grown guys have a high-school-boy attitude toward strange big-city restaurants and make themselves miserable. And that's silly.

Guests and Hosts

The business of being a host and being a guest can be tricky.

Being a guest ranges all the way from a drink at the local bar to drinks at someone's club to luncheon to dinner to a weekend at his home. Sometimes a point of escalation arrives when a man's wife gets involved. I don't want this last sentence to be misconstrued. I mean it in the most innocent way. (Hell, if a man's wife gets involved in *other* than an innocent way, there's no way I can give you advice in this book.)

Anyway, as long as it's just business-person-to-business-person, a "thank you" letter is good enough. Of course, if a fellow lends you his boat and captain for a weekend of fishing, the best thing is to find him a case of scotch. (Your host, not the captain.) The same to the senior vice-president or whoever decides to fly you around in his company's Lear Jet, providing Johnnie Walker Black Label and jet fuel aren't in short supply at the time (as this is written, many things are!).

If you're in any way involved with a man's *home* (and that includes his boat), then, chances are, you will have a hostess as well as a host. The easiest "thanks" is the flower routine. But you may want to be bit more personal, in which case you buy them the latest novel or, if you feel lavish or have had more than an evening's hospitality, a "coffee table" book. (Ask your bookdealer what the newest coffee table book is. He'll tell you.) If they're wine nuts, buy wine. If they're golf nuts, buy golf balls. Anyway, try to look as though you *thought* about the gift.

You *do* tip your hosts' employees when you've been a house or yacht guest. You don't tip their pilot. If their pilot has been flying you all over, send him a bottle of scotch. (Don't include a note which asks him not to drink it while he's flying. Pilots can be stuffy and easily hurt.)

In a home, you tip a maid or cook or whoever runs the house other than your hostess, but do it when no one is looking. Everyone knows you're tipping the servants, but it's better to do it discreetly. On a boat, about $20 a day is right for the captain. And if they have stewards and other help, give additional smaller tips. Never think of being a house-boat-plane guest as "saving dough." It's invariably as expensive as staying at a hotel.

Final note for houseguests: Use your credit card when making long-distance phone calls. It's amazing how a bunch of three-dollar calls can make you look like a crumb when your hostess checks the phone bill two weeks after you've left. She's bound to tell her husband.

About being a country-club guest: there used to be an old rule about "never inviting someone to be a guest at your club unless he was the kind of person you could propose for membership." That rule has faded fast, and today there are guys who invite business guests to their clubs whom they wouldn't invite to a public restaurant without being embarrassed. Nevertheless, assume that the old rule applies and that you are a club guest who behaves like a prospective member. Don't utter any criticism of the club, and if someone is rude to you, ignore it. Don't get bombed. Don't overstate your golf handicap. And before you order something, ask your host . . . even if it's to make a phone call. If the club is cruddy (and there are hundreds of cruddy country clubs around), behave with extra courtesy and avoid the possibilities of a drunken dinner with people you'd rather dodge by stating *early* that you have to be elsewhere for dinner. You can get the drift of things quickly. Don't dawdle if you want to get out right after your round of golf. If you're stuck, if you *must* stay for dinner, don't assume that hoisting a few drinks will make it easier for you. On the contrary. You'll probably get truthful (meaning rude) if you're slightly high. So, the cardinal rule is stay *sober*.

When you're invited to a famous restaurant and you suspect that *your* status in the restaurant is better than your host's status in the restaurant, offer to make the reservation for both of you. This way you won't end up sitting with the peasantry out there in Siberia, where the restaurant was going to seat your host; in addition, you'll protect your own precious "status" table.

If you pull this stunt as a guest, be sure to tip the maitre d' out of *your* pocket while your host isn't looking. If you couldn't con your host into letting you make the reservation, get to the restaurant fifteen minutes early and do your magic act with the maitre d'. If it's at all possible, he'll place you "right," after showing shock and saying, "But

Mr. Allardyce, I didn't know that Mr. Coward was bringing *you!*"

About "status" tables, no matter how many people tell you that doesn't matter and that their analysts have assured them that worrying about restaurant placement is a sign of insecurity, they're talking rot! There *are* "status" tables in every good restaurant, luncheon club, etc., and they *do* matter, unless you're the present or former governor of the state or Nelson Rockefeller or both. Human beings are achievement conscious and like to be associated with achievers . . . even if only geographically. In Russia it matters how many phones you have on your desk and which colors the phones are. It is perfectly understandable that a man or woman would want to protect his or her cherished status table in a restaurant without backsliding into the (sob) inferior position of a nonhabitué.

Of course if your host is better known than you are in a restaurant, goodie for you. I know more fellows who get invited to lunch and then quickly (when asked their choice) state the famous restaurant they know their prospective host usually frequents. Ever onward and upward! One of the signs of growing security is when the people at "good" tables around you begin to look crummy to you. Believe me, they haven't changed. *You* have. It's just that way back there, when they looked glamorous to you, they were already crummy, but you didn't know it!

I mentioned all the guest problems before I spoke of hostmanship because it is easy to be a host once you know a guest's problems. Just look at the above and reverse the roles.

Of course, I can't expect *you* to know if your own golf club is cruddy, but look at it this way: if you've occasionally felt that you've outgrown your club and would rather join a "better" club, then your golf club is probably cruddy.

Being a host at your home, the main trick is to *leave a guest alone*, to let him live as he wishes, *without neglecting him*. Give him every facility, from Kleenex to booze, from cigars to reading matter. Tell him when you generally eat. But don't force any issues. If it's a strain to have breakfast sent to his room on a tray, tell him that breakfast is anytime between seven and nine. Just don't regiment him. The best kind of hosts are those who arrange for a separate phone line for the guest room. That's true privacy.

As a rule, an invitation of more than three days is a bit of a push. Don't stretch things.

All of the above is needless advice if you're loaded with guest rooms and servants, because good servants can be your best hosts. But most of us lack such lavish trappings.

Entertaining guests from abroad. Unless they've been to your town many, many times, show them your home city, town, or village, but don't stress the civic institutions. No one is too impressed with stadiums or bank buildings. Show them your history. Show them the things which you, in moments of complete sentimentality, consider to be your favorite places. Take them out into the Indiana countryside or the foothills of the Rockies or Governor's Island (if you're in Indianapolis, Denver, or New York respectively). Foreigners are fascinated with American *history*. They like our heritage of pioneering and Indian fighting and gold prospecting and plantation life. Show them these things rather than the revolving rooftop restaurant overlooking glorious downtown Pottsville.

Don't kid yourself. Being a guest is often a lot tougher than being a host. These days it's not always true that those who *sell* are hosts and those who *buy* are guests. In fact, the most difficult kind of host is the fellow whom you need but who (for various reasons of his own) drags you into *his* bailiwick and becomes your host. It happens more and more. The big-time financial firms do it. The heavy industry fellows do it. Anyway, it's the new kind of guestmanship: how to be a guest of someone whom you're trying to sell something to.

The trick is not to lose sight of the thing you're trying to sell. If whatever you're offering is really first class, then being a guest shouldn't disturb you. Just accept hospitality the way you would when it's not a question of business and render the usual courtesies.

The Cardplayer

I lay no claim to Grand-Master ranking as a bridge player or even to a second income from poker winnings. However, I've noticed that there are certain psychological advantages to properly handling the preambles of any card game.

The thing which makes opponents quake more than any other (before getting down to the nitty-gritty of actual play) is shuffling and dealing. When a man shuffles and deals with *style*, everyone raises small-craft warnings at the table. Okay, if he's a dumb player, he'll probably lose anyway. But why not "spook" your opponent right at the start? It might even fluster him into an error. The old one-upmanship game.

So practice shuffling and dealing with style and flourish. Get some old-timer to show you how. Then shuffle, zzzip-zzip-zip and deal 'em out at a lightning rate. Finally, fan out your card hand with one flick of the thumb. Kill time on plane trips practicing.

The Car

What car should you wear?

That's right—wear. It's true you know, you put yourself into a car the way you put yourself into clothes. People look at you and they see your head and maybe your hands on the steering wheel, and that's exactly what they see of you when you're dressed. The rest is car. And they get an impression. They make judgments about your taste. Again, it's a matter of style.

Now, in the early Fifties it was very *inside* to drive a sports car (and we're talking about grown men, not kids). Other men one-upped the neighbors with a Caddy convertible or a maroon Buick sedan, but you, the grand avant-gardist of the country-club set, drove an **XK 120 Jag** or an **MGTC** or, *Bon Giorno, Dottre* . . . , a Ferrari.

Fine—even for most of the Sixties.

But now we're in the Seventies, and, *sic transit*, the sports car is no longer the inside toy for grownups. It has become the status gimmick of locks-in-the-wind youth. Good for them. Good luck to them. Let *them* try to find a mechanic who knows the inside of a Weber carburetor or fathoms the ignition on a British "sporty" engine, particularly on Saturday night or Sunday night. Sports cars break down only on Saturday nights or Sunday nights. It's a point of honor. ("Well"—scratch-of-the-head, scratch-of-the-head—"the only guy who knows these foreign things is Jack Carolinella an' he lives over in Brickville an' Sunday nights he's usually loaded. Anyways, parts have to come in from New York by air, I 'magine.")

The plain fact is that the small European sports car is just no longer as dashing as it was. Except a Ferrari. That's *always* dashing.

So, it's back to the station wagon (or, if gasoline remains a problem, one of the simple compacts). But *not*, please God, with the tapestry or gold- and silver-flecked interiors. The only way to get the car makers to build simple interiors, smarter interiors, is to declare a stubborn "No!" to motel decor.

But if you've outgrown a sports car and you're not satisfied with a domestic car and you've always longed for a Rolls or Bentley or Mercedes, go ahead! It's not as expensive as you fear—no more, say, than a medium-sized cabin cruiser. You've only got one life, baby. You deserve it. It will give you that zing feeling the kids get out of their sports cars. But in a grown-up way.

If you do drive a "stock" American car, though, why not dress it up a little by at least sporting some club badges? Surely you belong to *some* club? Or write for membership to one of the foreign auto clubs. They'll be happy to sell you a membership and the cost is slight. How does Auto Club of Morocco sound? Snazzy? Then why not? But don't just buy ersatz medallions in some novelty store and slap 'em on the front. That's tacky. Also, if you have a station wagon, you can paint the name of your country house on the side, discreetly, or of your boat. It's a minor manifestation of snobbery, but again, why not? Nothing wrong with painted initials, either . . . if they are discreet, remember. But crests? Well. . . .

If you're still bitten by the sports-car bug, do join the Sports Car Club of America. They have a great badge and you can read in their magazine all about who skidded off which track last month. An additional bit of inside poop; it's a fact that an SCCA badge on a stock car makes you look as if you have a McLaren race car tucked away somewhere. Very few race drivers, you know, choose small sports cars for everyday driving. Why? Well, for one thing, most of them are too lazy to shift gears when they don't have to.

There is, by the way, another trick to be learned from sports-car drivers—a *stylish* way to *drive* a car. Ridiculous? Well, I'm an ex–race driver, which qualifies me to point out a thing or two. Just watch the race drivers. They lean way back. Their arms are almost straight to the steering wheel. They drive at arm's length. Their seats are even built to recline. They look lazy and relaxed, although they're anything but.

Great athletes set the style for every sport, and driving is a sport, as coordinated and cerebral as golf, though a bit more murderous. Anyway, you should think of driving as a sport and concentrate, as if you were on the fairway. *And you should imitate the style of the pros.*

Why do the pros affect the arms-length way of driving? Because you can control the wheel more easily at arms length. Try it. Get right up to the wheel and hug it. Then see how quickly you can turn it through a full revolution, right or left. Tough, eh? Then move the seat back. Get away from the wheel and hold it at "nine o'clock" and "three o'clock" and try the same thing. Much easier? Right.

In driving, the *stylish* way is the *safe* way. It makes it a bit tough on the rear-seat passenger with long legs, but explain the whole thing to him. He'll give you a vinegary sort of smile and suffer in silence.

Barflies

Drinking alone at a strange bar is an American ordeal. Somehow you don't see too much of it in Europe. They've got pubs in England where friends converge and everyone gabs with everyone. In France and Italy the locals guzzle at outdoor café tables and it's much friendlier.

But in America, business guys arrive in a strange town and check into a motel or hotel and then there's nothing to do so we drift to a bar. It's a pretty grim ritual. You find your place and order your drink and then . . . nothing. If you start talking to your neighbor, chances are he won't be a charmer. The bartender is not about to enter into philosophical discourse. He's seen the same Bogart movies you have. You can't try "Give me one for my baby and one more for the road" on him. That's 1930s and he'll have none of it. In fact, the self-pitying romantic drunk is woefully out of fashion.

So have your drink, if you want a drink, and then cut out. The longer you stay there drinking, the less the likelihood of your enjoying yourself.

Somehow the American bar has become an unfriendly and noncommunicative place.

So drink and leave. If you want action, look for it elsewhere. If not, go back to the room and turn on the T.V.

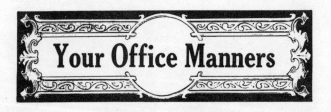

Your Office Manners

The Golden Rule —
Keep It Simple

The Office

I hereby announce the end, the finale, the demise, of the desk as a fortress. The idea of one man behind the desk and another man in front of it, of bully and victim, of ruler and subject is over. A desk is a place where an executive writes papers, examines papers, stores papers. Period.

Any man who uses his desk as a Maginot line deserves what the Maginot line got.

If a man gives you the desk routine, finesse him. Don't accept the chair he designates. Keep walking around so you can look *down* at him. Tell him you think better on your feet. Walk up to his wall and examine his plaques and look back at him over your shoulder. Or take another chair and move it around to the side of his desk, so he has to swivel. Move right up to his desk, opposite him, and lean on it as he does, so that you assume the same posture of attack. Drive him nuts. He deserves it.

An executive should leave his desk when you enter his office and wave you to a couch or to a small group of armchairs or to a meeting table. There should be an informal discussion area in each executive office where you can talk man-to-man, rather than boss to inferior or buyer to salesman-supplicant.

The ideal executive office, then, needs both a private "working" area and a neutral "meeting" area.

By the way, the executive who implies that he is mightily busy and is "squeezing you in" is a rude bastard. Chances are that if you allow him to get away with it, you'll never be able to present your case to receptive ears anyway. And chances are it doesn't matter. An ill-mannered businessman is usually incompetent.

The real killers are all charmers.

The Phone

Of course you've got a secretary. But you've also got a finger. Use it to dial your own calls. It's faster. It's flattering.

If you're talking to a subordinate, treat him as an equal. Tell him that you hope you're not interrupting. Ask him if he can spare a moment to step into your office. If he's in a meeting, ask him to call you when he gets a chance.

Of course, I realize the "him" may be a "her." In that case, all the rules stay the same. Don't treat businesswomen as if they are tender flowers. Treat them as teammates.

If you're using your secretary to place your call because you don't know a phone number or if you're placing a person-to-person long-distance call, make sure your secretary puts you on the second *before* your man gets on the phone.

You know what it feels like to be kept waiting while the caller takes his good old time picking up the phone. If someone has the habit of doing it to you, tell his secretary, gently, that you've got the devil of a busy office and would she call you back when her boss is ready to talk. She'll get the hint. Or simply hang up a few times and say that you must have been cut off. By the time her boss has picked up the phone several times without having you on the other end, she'll make darn sure that she never again keeps either one of you dangling.

There is a special world of long-distance and information operators. They must be spoken to slowly and distinctly and sort of led along, like children. If you are asking for the Bruce Plimsoll Corporation, explain that it might be listed under B or P. Operators are very sheltered people and you must demonstrate patience, restraint, and your best scoutmaster instincts.

For instance, suppose you say, "Operator, I want to call Paris." Well, that's no good. No good at all. She'll say: "I'll get Texas information." Serves you right.

Try this: "Operator, an *overseas* call to Paris."

By the way, it's better to direct-dial domestic long-distance calls. You can get information directly, you know: area code plus 555-1212. Forget person-to-person. If he's not in, might as well leave word directly at his office. It may cost a bit, but you can have a chat with his secretary. All secretaries love talking long-distance. Gives them a sense of adventure. Any long-distance caller is their special person. They'll get their boss to call back first chance, and you'll get a nice reception on future calls or visits.

Teach your children phone manners. "Who's calling him, please?" "I'll be glad to take your number." As it should be done. There's nothing worse than a teenager giving you the thug treatment:

"Is this the Thompson residence?"

"Yeah."

"Mr. Thompson, please."

"Not here."

"Where is Mr. Thompson?"

"Out."

"Can I leave word for him?"

"Guess so."

"All right, please tell him—"

"Wait a minnit. I'll get a pencil."

Makes the caller feel rejected and angry. No need for it.

One final bit of advice: Ask your secretary to tell people *exactly* why you can't answer the phone. None of that, "He's tied up" business. Rather: "He's got a number of people in his office." Or, "He's in the middle of a board meeting." Or, "He's stepped out for a few minutes." (Meaning that nature called. Don't let her carry things too far, though. No need for her to say, "He's got a real bad case of diarrhea this morning.")

The Business Letter

The business letter just may be obsolete. The telephone is gradually doing it in. The phone is fast and it is personal. Telephone service can be irritating but the mails can be maddening. In New York, many businessmen have given up on the mails for important correspondence; they rely on messengers. Telegrams and cables are also fast if you must put it "on the record." The need for speed and efficiency has also spawned the handwritten memo with built-in carbons. Longhand notes also eliminate the need for secretaries. Many large firms use typing pools, expert at mishearing, misinterpreting, and misspelling your dictaphone discs or recorder tapes.

Still, there are times when the business letter is unavoidable (if you have to have something reasonably formal in writing, for their files and yours, or there are details or instructions or legal matters to convey). But please, please, *please*, cut out all that unnecessary junk people stick into business letters, all that old-fashioned "business-ese." Be modern, crisp, efficient.

For example, instead of,

Dear Mr. Trumbull:

I am in receipt of your letter of August 3 and wish to inform you that the materials you requested are presently at hand and will be forwarded to you via the route you were kind enough to specify.

try the streamlined way:

Dear Mr. Trumbull:

Your order will be shipped Thursday, the 27th, via Railway Express.

In short, be short. Tell them what you want to tell them just as if you were talking on the phone. You wouldn't sign your letter, "Your obedient servant," would you? So cut out all the other Victorian nonsense as well. No more "you were kind enough" or "thanks for your consideration" or references to yourself as "the writer" or "the undersigned."

If you do have a mass of details, have them typed on a formal second sheet and attach them to a short covering letter. Much easier for the other side to handle, copy, and distribute.

If you have legalese to forward, however, do *not* simplify, unless you yourself have practiced law. Leave all the lumpy, pompous, convoluted language intact. Lawyers are jealous guardians of their voodoo and to tangle with their incantations is to invite dire afflictions.

If your letter is to a friend, then close with "Kindest personal regards" or "Best wishes to Kate" (his wife, we trust, not his secretary) or some other friendly word. Or, better yet, do a handwritten P.S. below your signature.

Another thing: unless your signature is hopelessly illegible, don't have your name typed. It's just more unnecessary formality. Ask your secretary to type only your job description, if it is needed.

A word about those office politicians who tell a guy something on the phone, then write him a covering letter "confirming our telephone conversation of this morning," then *blind* copy the whole damn thing to his boss and your boss and lord knows who else's boss. Well, maybe it works and he is "safe" if there is a goof-up, but successful executives spend their time moving ahead, not covering their tracks. Seldom will anyone trot out an old letter, Watergate-style, and confront an associate with it. Six months after that blind copy, no one's tail can be saved by proving you "were right," because you will be judged on a lot more than an old letter.

When writing business letters abroad, remember to simplify. And we mean *simplify*. Use basic English, strictly first-grade-reader, and give them a chance. Imagine a French secretary trying to translate "low profile" for her boss! Even the British may not comprehend our business English, for theirs can be different; to them, for example, "volume" means "turnover" and "stocks" are "shares." So forget the business page lingo and write like a dum-dum.

There is one other time when only a letter will serve: when sending congratulations. Most people are better off putting their gush on paper. It's damnably hard to say to someone on the phone, "Warmest congratulations on winning the magnificent award, Henry. No one deserved such

recognition more than you." So don't phone—
write.

But, once again, keeping it short will keep it
sounding sincere. Don't overdo it. Most people who
have been profiled in newspapers and magazines or
who have been promoted or won awards feel
slightly embarrassed about it all, and once they've
read the company's P.R. handouts, they begin to
wonder if they even deserved the damn things.
They are quick to brush off anything that sounds
like flattery. A praise letter should be like one of
those affectionate fist-pokes on the arm: light,
chummy, and quick.

How to Talk to One's Secretary and to Someone Else's Secretary

Politely. Very politely. Always. It's the only way.

Business Cards

There's the fellow who barely nods "glad to meet you" before he's snapped out a business card. And the one who disdainfully tells you he has given up carrying cards; the world should recognize him *instanter*. There's also the man who tells you, "I really never carry a card . . . but I guess I've got one here somewhere." He fumbles through his wallet, then hands you a dog-eared card penciled with the list of groceries his wife asked him to pick up five months before.

Well, you *should* have cards, neat and accessible. And not just one kind, but two. You should carry personal cards as well as business cards. Not crucial, we know, and fallen into neglect, but personal cards are a polished accompaniment to flowers and other gifts, including business gifts. They are most handy and—well, personal—when you want to give someone your home address and phone number. Since a personal card just states your name—nothing else—in that case you *write them* on the card just before handing it over.

Your business card, of course, has your title as well as your name, and the name, address, and phone number of your company. Most corporations insist upon a standard company-wide format for their cards, and you can't do much about it. Unless you reach the top. In that case, we hope you insist upon some style in the design of your company's cards. A change of type face away from the stereotype face.

Some corporate presidents do vary the corporate design for their own cards. One president we know has just his name printed on his business cards, plus the symbol of his corporation. The symbol, it is true, is internationally recognizable, but it does seem a trifle un-humble. Even presidents can be pushy, you know, because unless you are the chief exec at GM, there's always a corporation bigger than yours.

On the other hand, if you are a *very* big shot, you could eliminate at least the title. After all, if you're Henry Ford, you don't have to explain your job at the Ford Motor Company.

It's dreary to be handed a business card within two minutes after the first "hello." Unless you are in Japan, where an immediate exchange of cards is ceremonial—more on that in our chapter on Japan —don't be in a hurry. Save the exchange of identifications for the *end* of a conversation. If you and the chap beside you in the airplane have struck up a well-martinied friendship, hand him your business card just before you land. This timing is especially desirable if he might be able to send some business your way. The suave approach is never to be too eager or anxious. Unhurried and unharried.

About the use of middle initials and family paraphernalia on business cards, opinions clash. Most true bigwigs are now passing up the twin middle initials or the "H. Stuart Montague Forsythe III" stuff. If you are sufficiently secure, Stuart Forsythe will do nicely. After all, who knows Robert McNamara's middle initial?

a lot of people

S.

When to Call Someone "Sir"

There are so many kinds of "sirs." There's the "sir" rendered by minor subordinates to the very superior. There's the "sir" bellowed out by an elder gentleman telling a young whippersnapper where he gets off: "Don't give me any of that nonsense, sir!" There's the business of being trapped in one's own strict up-draggin' and calling everybody of one's father's generation "sir." There's the moment when one feels cowed by a state trooper and one calls him "sir"—although he'll hand out the ticket anyway.

In business, however, after a certain age and a certain level of success, "sir" should be reserved only for very senior officers, so senior they are poised for a pension. Most modern-day upper-level executives are quite young and "sir"-ing them only creates unnecessary barriers. It's as antiquated as the old "initial" game, when fellows in business were called "H.R." or "J.M." That came out of the family business days when privately owned corporations had a slew of sons or cousins all bearing the same last name and one had to define which was which Fotheringill. It's faded fast, and so has the need for the deferential "sir."

We can think of one exception. When introduced to a senior government official, such as a cabinet member, it might be well to use "sir" at least at your first meeting. He may be near your own age, but it's an homage you can pay to power.

In Writing

Long before you meet a guy face to face, you may meet him by mail. And by mail he may be a fatuous ass, a pompous fuddy-duddy, a prissy prig. Which may not be true at all. It's just that his letter might have been fatuous, pompous, or prissy. People can get very strange when they pick up a pen or dictaphone. Proper and defensive, assuming a pose, the way they stiffen when having their picture taken. Try to be natural when you write or dictate a letter, to sound as you would in conversation.

Other unnecessary stuffiness: you get a personal letter about a personal matter, such as a charity deal or a golf game or your son's graduation, and the darn thing is on a corporate letterhead with "Office of the Vice-President in Charge of Sales" in the left-hand corner and "Malcolm D. Connors III" under the scribbled "Mal." For heaven's sake, if you're a V.P. and a fairly big shot, you don't need to display your full-dress battle ribbons to say: "Meet you at eleven on Saturday and give my best to Helen."

Have some nice small "private" stationery printed. On top have your first and last name only.

No real big-timer needs initials. After all, it's
Dwight Eisenhower, Richard Nixon, Gregory Peck,
Charles Lindbergh. Who the hell cares about initials? If you feel like a big-timer, act like one.
About the Jr. and III game, use it only if your
pater or pater's pater is alive. And don't bother
printing the address. Just say "Henry Axelgrief" on
top in small block letters, embossed. Your secretary can type in the address over the date. That
way you can write from your house, your yacht,
your summer estate, your ranch outside Buenos
Aires, or your Lear Jet without changing stationery. Also, on your private letterhead ask your secretary to skip the initial routine in the lower left
corner. It's too "businessy." *Don't* have your name
typed under your signature either. Just sign. They'll
know who it is from by looking at the top of the
letter. If you really want to personalize, *hand-write*
the "Dear Tom" or "Dear Herman." It's a bit
British-affected, but you'd be surprised how many
people like it.

   For that matter, there are tons of ways of writing in a very personal manner.

   For instance: Have $4\frac{1}{4}''$ by $5\frac{1}{4}''$ cards made
with your name *embossed* on top. Then write your
notes by hand. All the "Thanks for lunch" and "It
was a great party" ones. It takes two minutes and
makes you look super. Your secretary can type the
envelope.

   Or have them print miniature-size legal pads,
the yellow-lined kind, about $8''$ by $5''$, with your
name on top in red. Then scribble your personal
message. You can even do it for many business
communications, like business thank yous. If you
must have copies, use the Xerox. It takes you two

seconds to scribble, the guy you're addressing is flattered silly that you're bothering to handwrite and your secretary is grateful.

"Yacht" type stationery with crossed burgees or "Aboard Yacht Goosefat" are rather scruffy, unless you own a legit, honest-to-goodness, captain-run, documented yacht. If it's just a nice 35' cabin cruiser or a juicy 35' ketch, you're really over-doing it a bit to put on yachting airs. Okay, so you're registered in Lloyd's, but so is everyone who wants to register his boat if she's over 30'.

Same goes for country homes. Unless you have an honest-to-goodness estate with curving drive-way and chauffeur and cook and butler and up-stairs maid, don't send out notes with "Grey Acres" or "Moist Bottom" printed on top. The address will do.

If you really value your privacy, just have your personal address printed on the back of your personal envelopes. No name.

If you're really a big-time entrepreneurial blockbuster, have the backs of your business enve-lopes printed with just your initials and the office address, with suite number, if necessary.

For instance:

22 West 55th Street
New York, N.Y. 10019

means "Nelson Rockefeller," even without the initials. That's that.

About signatures: It's getting to be more and more "in" to sign legibly. The days of illegible signatures (to show that you whip off *thousands* of documents each day) are fading.

When you've been on a business trip and everyone has poured champagne all over you and you've had *male* hosts, why not use the flight back to handwrite your thank yous on airline stationery? No harm. People feel that you're thinking about their hospitality while you're flying home. If you've had *female* hosting, send flowers *before* you leave town and write your own card. Trouble with telegraphed flowers is that your thank you may be written for you by a teenager with acne'd handwriting.

Finally, telegrams and cablegrams are extra special. Night letters are cheap and equally effective. And don't use telegraphese in personal telegrams or cables. None of this "DINNER GREAT THANKS HENRY" stuff. Go the whole route. "DEAR MARGIE AND BOB LOVED HAVING DINNER WITH YOU AND MEETING YOUR GREAT KIDS HOPING TO SEE YOU SOON IN LAUDERDALE ALL BEST AS EVER HENRY." What the hell, you've got twenty-five words in night letters. Go for broke, Marmaduke!

Women in Business

Talking to a woman in business is, well, pretty much like talking to a man in business. Your approach will depend on her job and your job, her charm and your charm, who's buying and who's selling. In other words, business as usual.

And that means just what you think it means —it's products and services you are buying and selling, not sex. Sure, you can be charming. You're also charming with a guy you want to do business with. But the heavy breathing and heavy leering is not only crummy, it is, in the case of a bright woman, totally ineffective. In fact, you stand a very good chance of lousing up everything.

Consider the opposite situation. A woman comes into your office on a business call. You're a pretty bright guy who knows what he's doing. If she pulls a *femme fatale* act, you might be flattered and tempted at first, but then you'd say to yourself, "Hell, she's trying to *con* me into this deal! I'm no patsy." After that you'd be suspicious.

It is just as much of an offense to a woman's intelligence to be approached that way. The day of

the big deal "waltzed in" by way of the couch is
over, now that women are becoming more of a
routine part of the business world. Business is
rough. No one can afford decisions based on libido.

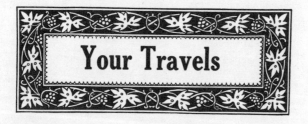

Your Travels

Fly Right!

The Trip

I realize that in this enlightened age the above title leads you to expect some words about "turning on." Uh uh. I mean to talk about, literally, the trip—business or pleasure. (Are there still pleasure trips, or do we manage to find a deduction even though we're 100 feet below surface, skindiving? "Well, you see, Mr. Tax Inspector, the only reason I took skindiving lessons is that everyone I could sell insurance to was down there, bubbling. Why else would I take scuba lessons? Think I'm a nut or something? Of *course* it's deductible!")

First of all, business or pleasure, we always pack too much. There isn't a one of us who hasn't come home with some of the same clean shirts we took away. Secondly, we pack *stupidly*.

Business trip. Two days. By plane. Wear one suit, pack one. Pack it in a zipper bag, the kind you carry on and hand to the hostess. Open up your spare shirt and *hang* it in the same bag, under the jacket. Your spare tie, ditto, on the same hanger. Make sure the suit you're wearing and the suit you're dragging can take the *same color shoes*, so you don't have to take a second pair. Underwear, PJs (bottoms only), and spare socks all go into your carry-on-stash-under-seat bag. More on that bag in the next episode.

Take along a raincoat (summer) with, if needed, a zip-out lining (winter).

Forget the hat. Business hats have had it, as I've said. If you're scared of getting your curls wet, stash a roll-up rain hat in your raincoat pocket.

Now you're carrying *everything* aboard and you can hustle for a taxi while the others are still waiting for their checked baggage. Airline hostesses get hernias this way, but you're ahead of the game.

You can get away with the carry-on game up to four days. After that, it gets a bit sticky. If you're staying the weekend, take along extra slacks (wear one pair and a blazer on the plane), and hang your sweaters under your suit jacket. If you have to take golf shoes or tennis shoes and racket, take an extra small carry-on bag. But don't try to carry on your golf bag. Also, remember you can stuff much into your raincoat pockets, like spare socks or underpants. Just be sure they don't fall out in the Hilton lobby.

If you're overseas, go ahead and check your bags. You have to go through customs anyway, and sometimes a friendly baggage carrier (well-tipped) can speed up the customs routine. We've found that the best kind of bag, if you *are* checking, is the big foldover hang-up case. Don't forget to carry your passport in your carry-on luggage, because you have to fill out immigration forms and who the hell remembers his passport number? You'll also need the passport for getting by the local gestapo when you land.

Especially for the bitchy-long trips, like to Tel Aviv or Tokyo, be sure to carry on your shaving gear. As you stumble off the old 747 after twenty hours on a plane, there may be eight people to kiss and hug you. And you don't want to look all stubbly and scruffy, do you, Ronald? Besides, it makes a better impression on the Immigration and Customs blokes when you look half decent.

More neat little tricks:

Store your socks in your shoes when you're packing for the longer hauls.

Take one of the knitted suits. It'll survive your ham-fisted packing.

You can wash your underpants in the sink in all European countries. They all have heated towel racks in their bathrooms and your dainties will dry overnight.

Do buy some clothes on trips abroad. Not that there are so many great things to buy, but they'll give you a worldly boost when they reappear in your closet back home. And they supply good lines like: "Oh, that shirt? Yes, it is rather nice. Picked it up on the Via Condotti last time over."

Warning, most European shoes will *kill* you. They usually make only one width. But the shops have very snazzy salesgirls. So you'll think the shoes fit because the salesgirl has pretty legs. But they won't. Fit, that is.

Tip: Joint called Asprey's in London has the best note pad for travel in the world. It's very flat. You'll love me for telling you. It's also the mark of the world traveler, and you *love* status symbols, don't you, Ernest?

Tip: If you want to cheer your foreign business associates, bring them gold *Cross* pens. They are status symbolic in *their* business crowd. Bring silver ones to Japan. In Japan all gold stuff is considered pushy.

Don't try bringing Cuban cigars from England or France. Our custom boys are very moralistic about Cuban cigars. You'll get the bamboo treatment after the water torture. For that matter, the Cubans are just as tough about American cigars. So if you get hijacked, don't try to sell your American cigars in Havana. They'll get very hot under their beards, the Cubans will.

We'll have more to say about what to wear abroad, but let it be noted here that many chic Europeans travel in turtlenecks, sports jackets, and slacks. You can *check into* the best hotels that way. They'll understand. But you shouldn't overdo it. They won't let you into the dining room in that same turtleneck. The Europeans are fairly stuffy about things sartorial, no matter what you hear about the swinging English, the *dolce vita* Italians, or the worldly French.

The Japanese are very formal, too, and if you overdo the casual stuff they may raise their eyebrows. Japan is tie-and-shirt country. Turtlenecks are okay for golf, but that's all.

Luggage

Since I fly all over the world—some 100,000 miles a year—to stay in touch with those who sell, make, buy, and wear my designs, I have become somewhat of a luggage expert.

Invariably accompanying me on the plane, at least for business trips, is a small, soft-sided canvas bag made by T. Anthony, the New York luggage shop. No doubt Mark Cross, Vuitton, and others purvey something similar. It has two side pouches and an open section in the middle. Under the seat it goes.

Into one pouch I have stashed my shaving gear, one set of clean underwear, my PJs, and socks. If my luggage is lost, at least I can shave and shower until my belongings have been winged back to me.

In the other pouch I put a flat, zippered leather folder or "envelope," empty and folded in half to fit easily into the pouch. Into the fold of this folder go whatever travel papers I might need —traveler's checks and passport usually. I even keep my ticket there, readily accessible, not bunching up my pockets. Behind the leather folder I put whatever business papers I have to take, sorted into manila folders.

The open section in the middle? Magazines, a paperback, smoking matter, and a pack of Klee-nex. Any quick-grab stuff.

When I get to my hotel, I take out the empty leather folder, which now becomes my briefcase. I stick into it whatever manila folders I will need for that day.

I find this beats the conventional hard-sided commuter briefcase, which just isn't big enough to hold toilet articles and clothes as well as papers. Much more streamlined this way.

To review. Tickets, passport? You know right where they are. Business stuff to study en route? You've got it with you. Shave before landing? Easy. Luggage lost for twenty-four hours? You can still smell clean.

By the way, in many good European hotels luggage does *not* accompany you to your room. The reception clerk shows you to your room and the baggage follows, maybe a good ten minutes later. You can't do the familiar American routine of getting things sorted out and hung up before heading for the phone. But this way you *can* un-pack your clean-up gear. If you're in the shower when the luggage finally arrives, it will only save you from tipping. Serves 'em right.

Flying There

I realize that most companies have strict rules about who flies first class and who goes to the back of the cabin, and that you may not as yet—fear not, the day will come—qualify for front rank. Some corporations, particularly when profits are, as they say, flat, require all to fly cheaply. Well, I say unless you're broke, flat broke—and maybe even if you are—*fly first class*. And if your firm won't ante up, pay the difference yourself.

Sure, I know all the arguments against first class. Particularly the one about "earning money while sitting on your bottom for a few hours."

No, it's not the steak or the champagne I'm thinking about. It's meeting other passengers who may be of help to you one day. And it's the frame of mind created by riding in style, the feeling of assurance it breeds. You arrive pitched for success. In short, it's a good investment.

Maybe you made it big long ago and no longer need connections or assurance. In that case you can fly economy class, but as for me, I'll take first class. *Basta.*

About the "right" time to fly. To the Orient, each trip is rough. It's a long flight. I think that the best suggestion I've heard is to be sure to arrive in

Japan between midnight and 7 A.M., because even the energetic Japanese won't pull you into an instant meeting at that unholy time. So you can get your breath back before you're asked to function. If you get to your hotel at 3 A.M. you can stall everyone and everything until, say, lunch that day. (What'a ya want, Harold, a rest cure? Then go to Philadelphia.)

But to Europe, there are two schools of thought. Some prefer leaving in the A.M., and that means, whether you fly over the Pole from the West Coast or from New York, Boston, or Washington, you blow a day. I am of the P.M. school. Leave about nine or ten from New York, after a pleasant dinner, and arrive in London or Amsterdam or Paris in the morning. No days lost.

That is, it makes sense *if* you can sleep on a plane. It's no fun to face a business day after thirty-six sleepless hours. If you have to do it, swear to yourself you'll take an afternoon snooze at the hotel; else you'll collapse over dinner, which could make your hosts feel unloved.

By the way, don't be too concerned about talk of jet lag. It's mainly talk, as you've probably found out for yourself by now. The body comes back in a hurry. The only thing I might suggest for those of you nearing—well, the mature years—is to bring your laxative.

Coming back to the U.S. from Europe always offers that nice "time surprise." You have a business breakfast at your hotel, arrive at the airport at noon and land in New York in time for cocktails and dinner. Going back it all works out *right*. Going there is not half the fun.

Which airline? Well, they're all good. When **going abroad, however, it's a good idea to fly on the** airline of the country you're visiting. You get a chance to acclimate yourself to the upcoming country, to hear its accents, to eat its foods, to flip through its magazines. If you are flying to Britain, you can read the London newspapers. You can read what Londoners are reading about British politics, sports, economics—and what Londoners are reading about *us*. You'd be surprised. The *Daily Express* has an absolutely vile little column about America which invariably plays up riots, murders, robberies, scandals, and all manner of disasters, natural and man-made. Their tabloids picture us in stereotypes. We are brash and pushy and violent. But calm down, Herman. They don't believe their papers any more than we do ours.

New York

For those of you who are startled by New York (and that includes a lot of New Yorkers), try looking at it this way: New York is a costume party, sometimes an evil costume party, but mostly just a funny costume party. It is the insecurity center of America, the place where more people try to con more people than anywhere else. Sometimes they succeed, because New York does not allow anyone to know anyone long enough to get the goods on them. Also, because New Yorkers are so busy doing their own con job, they haven't the energy to analyze someone else's.

There are other insecurity areas in our country, like Beverly Hills, Palm Springs, Palm Beach, Southampton. But these are only branch offices. The corporate headquarters is New York.

First and foremost: Don't let it worry you. If you're a visitor, observe it and laugh. If you're a New Yorker, just make sure you've got enough money. It's the only way to feel secure in New York.

Maybe you live elsewhere and come to New York two, three, five times a year and you still find it somewhat baffling. Maybe this will help you get a handle on it. (I'll only speak about the core,

the part which sets the mood for most visitors.)
Let's dissect.

Maybe you live in Indianapolis and come
into the big city two, three, five times a year and
you still find it somewhat baffling. Maybe this will
help you get a handle on it.

Let's dissect.

Third Avenue. That's the Executive Suite of
Insecurity, Inc. It's a haven for pretense, because
most of the Third Avenue people are flat broke.
Their boozing and eating joints are super ham-
burger hangouts (deluxe oversize overtrimmed
hamburgers, but hamburgers nonetheless) and
beer parlors (imported premium beers, but beers
nonetheless). Each one of these joints has an elab-
orate structure, usually built around minor celebrities and good press agents. Once in a while Jackie
Onassis or some other *real* celeb stops by to slum.
Then the press agents go mad. Anyone over thirty
who hangs out regularly on Third Avenue is usually
a failure with curly hair, a Mongol moustache, and
the latest in fake European gear. Snakeskin shirts
are in? They wear snakeskin shirts. Red velvet
boots? Red velvet boots. There are dozens of boutiques all along the Avenue which go bankrupt and
reopen, go bankrupt and reopen. They usually
have cute sexy names like Three Balls or Fagazine,
names to vomit from. They sell homemade gar-
bage or imports from Europe's bad boutiques. The
Third Avenue Insecures are fickle; they run after
the latest thing like sheep, and if a boutique falls
two days behind the latest gimmick, it gets frozen
out.

At night, many Third Avenue Insies move
over to the singles bars on Second and First Ave-
nues, where they drink more beer and pee more

and flirt with Brooklyn and Queens girls and girls
from Cleveland and Milwaukee, all of whom wear
the latest nonsense and take the pill and speak
meaningfully in Brooklyn, Queens, Cleveland, and
Milwaukee accents. Yes, there's pot. Yes, they
sometimes get laid. No, they don't have a good
time. It's all too frantic, because everybody is so
busy looking and acting "in" and trying to stay
cool, that nobody laughs out loud and has a ball.

Sometimes, the Third Avenuers stand in line
for hours at their Third Avenue movie houses
which are very small and play very "in" movies.
These long waiting lines have nothing to do with
the movie inside. The movie is the kind that
"ought" to be seen because it's "meaningful" and
"relevant" (screwing, pot, youth vs. age, black vs.
white), but most of all, the movie lines are freak
fashion shows and the hour or so spent on the side-
walk is a Third Avenue social gala. See the boy in
the two pigtails with the Moroccan pimp's pants
and the red turban! See the girl with the shaved
head and the First World War Cavalry tunic!
Smashing? Smashing! Right on!

From there, New York puffs its way toward
other peaks.

Lexington Avenue. Lex is Third Avenue with
inflation, both in price and age. There are more
marrieds, more sophistication, better clothes in the
boutiques, and better food in the eateries. But the
people are still playing a role, and look more tired
doing it.

Both Third and Lexington pivot around
Bloomingdale's and Alexander's. Bloomies is a
dear, solid, old store, a mainstay of New York
which plays footsies with the Third Avenue and
Lexington Avenue freaks, but makes its money on

middle-class New Yorkers with delusions of chic. Everyone shopping in Bloomingdale's looks a bit like the old Elaine May - Mike Nichols characters, and talks a little like them too. Bloomingdale's is something like a nice old synagogue with a discothèque in the annex. You never know if they're coming in to pray or to dance. It's a really great store, and knows the score. If they sometimes put on airs, it's not because they really mean it.

Alexander's is a mass discount store with an enormous capacity for fashion opportunism. They swing, and I mean swing. Whatever evil new fashion may emerge from France or Britain or Italy, Alexander's has it, and has it for *less*. In between the freak customers are pleasant old women looking for warm woolies for their husbands. It's all there, from champagne at Dr. Pepper prices to flowered housedresses for the varicose-vein set.

Park Avenue. Upward and onward. Park Avenue is . . . Park Avenue. What can I tell you? No boutiques or department stores. Just offices and, above 59th Street, apartments. Park Avenue apartments. But whenever you're super impressed, think of it this way: count all the hundreds of big apartment houses on each side of Park Avenue and multiply by the number of apartments and the number of people who seem to be able to afford each one. Suddenly "exclusive" Park Avenue doesn't look so exclusive anymore. Suddenly you realize that there are probably more people living on Park Avenue than the total population of most medium-sized towns.

Madison. Now we're getting into real stuff, real respectable stuff. Madison truly is a luxury shopping street, from about 50th Street up, with the money bulge concentrated in the 60s and low

70s. But though the shoppers themselves seem pretty glamorous, in truth they're about as miserable as their brethren on Third and Lex. Again, mostly costume party. It's more "upper," it's a bit more mature (age, not attitude), and it's substantially more expensive. But it's the same silly game. Any spring or fall Saturday on Madison Avenue will show you the Madison Avenue mambo, which consists of strollers wandering into the galleries where they will never buy a painting, window shopping the clothes boutiques so they will know what to buy at Alexander's, and stopping where they auction stuff most people can't afford (most people attending the auctions, that is). Whereas Third and Lex fashions are Paris Left Bank and London Chelsea, Madison fashions are Paris Right Bank and London Mayfair. Anything but America, which is considered beneath the notice of most New Yorkers. Eventually you come to the conclusion that New York is only administratively part of America. It is emotionally part of Europe.

Fifth Avenue. Fifth is a fading business street, as the junk shops ("Genuine Swiss watches, $7.95 and up") swarm in on Saks, and fine specialty shops are replaced by Abyssinian Airways offices.

But above 59th, Fifth is a super exclusive residential street. In that respect, Fifth Avenue is what Park Avenue pretends to be.

Restaurant life. I'll discuss only the top few. The rest are like restaurants anywhere else in America.

"21." Mainly big business, big sports, and the established entertainers. There are no fashion rules. You dress at "21" as you would in any top restau-

rant in Chicago or Dallas. In fact, many of its best clients are very much from Chicago and Dallas. "21" is not really "chic" in the jet-set sense. Chairmen of the boards of big Western industrial corporations who would be sniffed at by jet-set headwaiters get the royal treatment at "21." It's an industry-oriented place. The celebrities you find there are usually of the John Wayne variety: old-timers, rich, conservative, huntin'- and shootin'- (and sometimes boozin'-) type celebs. Don't let "21" scare you. It has a mass of tables (although there are only a few "in" areas) and you can always get seated. It's not *overly* expensive. Just expensive. They have a man at the desk when you walk in. He's not there to keep you out (unless you're wearing blue jeans). He's there to greet you if you're *somebody*. He'll even greet nobodies if he's known them long enough. In fact, "21" has certain nobody clients who've gone there for thirty years and have become "21"-bodies, a special breed of New Yorker. "21" is loyal to its old clients, no matter who they are. The food is rough and ready, but good. Do make reservations, not that it matters from the point of view of where you sit, but it does get you seated fast in case they're crowded. Sometimes the barflies are more interesting than the diners. Members of the jet set are not "21"ers. It's too American for them. And too solid.

La Grenouille, La Caravelle, Côte Basque, Lafayette. These are the jet-set restaurants, the insider's places for those who do the London-Rome-Marbella-St. Moritz-Palm Beach-Southampton circuit. They all have superb food, and they are all gossip-shooting galleries within the jet-set preserve. There are "good" and "bad" tables in

all of them, and there's no way of immediately tipping your way into the "good" side. There are only
two reasons to go to these places: superb cuisine—
really great, great cooking—or international social
climbing. Settle for the cooking. If you want to
keep score of who ate at which one, read *WWD*
(*Women's Wear Daily*). I know I sound like I'm
kidding, but actually it's the biggest restaurant
gossip column in New York. (There's also Suzy,
the columnist in the *News*, and Eugenia Sheppard
in the *Post*. More about that later.) All these restaurants are run by master restaurateurs, usually
French. They're absolute perfectionists. So are the
waiters, also French. They're all *lovely* restaurants,
physically charming, covered with fresh flowers
(which cost thousands per year) and they'd all die
on their feet if they weren't heavily populated by
beautiful women in beautiful clothes, the *Vogue-
Bazaar-Town & Country* untouchables. Movie
actresses? Only a few. The top ones. No starlets,
please, and no minor TV types. It all sounds for-
bidding, but it isn't if you don't allow yourself to
get dented by the "who sits where?" game. Make a
reservation and they'll stick to it. If you don't sit
next to the Duchess of Windsor, that's your tough
luck. What did you expect, Mortimer? But what
you don't know won't hurt you. And if you've got
fast and sneaky eyes, and you're noticing things,
you'll see where the duchesses sit. Then go back
often and tip well. Maybe you'll get promoted,
eventually. Hint around. Say that you prefer the
light in the front room.

What to wear? As we said about "21"—tie,
shirt, suit . . . the usual restaurant paraphernalia.
Except La Grenouille, where at lunch you can wear

the right sort of turtleneck (terribly expensive) under your jacket or perhaps even a velveteen vest suit over a silk dot shirt. (On the other hand, I doubt if any of you own a velveteen vest suit. I don't. Frankly, I'd feel like a nut walking around in velveteen.)

A few other in spots: *Orsini's*. Very jet-set. The Onassises courted there. Here, too, you can wear the right sort of turtleneck (at lunch). *The Running Footman*. Very in, but not too pretentious. Good tweed jacket place. *Veddy* British. *L'Aiglon*. The oldest existing French (or "continental," which is mostly French) restaurant, where I last saw Noel Coward in New York.

Two hotels have socially "acceptable" eating places. The Plaza (Oak Room) and the St. Regis (Oak Room and King Cole Bar). Both are tie-and-shirt places and there are no real "in" and "out"— that is, status and nonstatus—tables. King Cole Bar has a minor "21" crowd with a famous ancient off-color story: The huge painting of King Cole on his throne (on the back wall) has two jesters who supposedly are making faces because the King has just, er, broken wind. Most King Cole regulars first heard that story the year of Pearl Harbor. But you go ahead and enjoy it now, hear?

Trader Vic's. I know it sounds silly, but dear old hick-haven, Trader Vic's, which looks like all the other T.V.'s and their imitations all over the U.S.A., is very "in"; at least the front rooms are, *on Sunday nights only*. The rest of the time it's just Trader Vic's with all the Polynesian bora-bora.

Nightspots. Very few, because New Yorkers have scuttled night life. The good ones are: *El Morocco*, a private club. Sorry. *Le Club*. A private club. Sorry. The *Carlisle Hotel Bar*. Bobby Short plays the piano and sings. Bobby (who is on the International Best-Dressed List) is the darling of those on the International Best-Dressed List. He rules a gloss crowd at crowded tables with a tender Cole Porter whip.

About the private night clubs. Eventually someone you know will take you there. The membership list is immense. Then make up your mind if you want to join. It's tough to join because they're so damned crowded. (Nothing to do with your social status. Many nonprominences belong.) It's also damned expensive. If you want to spend the money, you'll get in. Just wait your turn. All private night clubs in New York start with a few selected people. But they can't exist that way. So they raise the initiation fee and open the door a bit. Then, zowie. They get swamped. And the joint no longer looks as good. Can't all be movie stars. Must also have a few druggists, provided they're *rich* druggists. Right?

Hotels. There are only a few smart hotels in New York. The rest are commercial joints with conventioneers. The moment you see the name tags with "D.L. Carter, Rockville Division" pinned on their jackets, it's all over.

Here are *the* hotels: *Plaza* (broken-down but prestigious). *St. Regis* (ditto). *Carlisle* (superb). *Pierre* (superb). *Regency* (not bad).

There are also second-rank excellences like the *Stanhope* (upper Fifth Avenue), the *Dorset*, the *Gotham*, the *Surrey*, the *Beekman*, and the *Drake*.

Despite its famous reputation, the *Waldorf* has unfortunately become just another commercial hotel. This does not include the Towers; mostly private apartments, they remain a super celeb haven at the very senior level.

Most sophisticated New Yorkers entertain at home. Chances are that unless your hosts are very formal (which you must know from being acquainted), you can get by with blazer and slacks, tie and shirt. If people say black tie, though, *wear* black tie.* If they take you to any one of the above restaurants, wear a dark suit, tie, and shirt—don't take chances—unless, again, the party is black tie. New York is the only major city in the world which is still black-tie-happy. London, Rome, Paris have long ago given up the whole thing.

If you want to entertain in New York, best hire a car and chauffeur to get you and your guests around. There are a zillion rental services, and your hotel, if it's a good one, will provide car and chauffeur and charge your account. It also braces your back when you drive up to strange restaurants.

Odds and ends.

The corner of New York I have described is a small corner. But it's the one usually written or talked about, the "chic" New York. There are many other New York worlds, like the Racquet Club–Darien commuters world or the "Street" (Wall, that is). If you deal with Wall Street on business, they'll probably take you to one of the commercial luxury restaurants like Four Seasons, Forum, etc. These are really not "in" places, although they're perfectly good, have excellent food

---

* And "black tie" means the quiet and underplayed sort of tuxedo I discussed earlier. Never, *never* a fancy-shmantzy one!

and service, and charge bombastic prices. But somehow they've never quite made it on the super pretentious jet-set circuit. So, if someone takes you to one of these, don't expect to see "inside" New York. Chances are the clientele is very nice and prosperous and all that, but not Suzy material.

New York theater. Unhappily, it is usually a bore. Most plays are third-rate and you've made a big effort for zilch. Use a broker (the hotel usually has one), and then call *Sardi's* and try to get a table at the front, so you can see actors. Curtain time is now 7:30 P.M., so you'll eat early (10:15). Because Sardi's is really actor-producer-director-playwright-composer country, no one else really counts. The only socialites who mean a damn at Sardi's are the ones who are theater hangers-on. Of course, Sardi's, like any other large restaurant, has a vast crowd of nobody clients who fill up two floors' worth of tables, but often you can be in luck and stare at Alec Guinness or Paul Newman or Hitchcock.

New York reading. "In" pages: Suzy (*Daily News*). Eugenia Sheppard (*Post*). Charlotte Curtis' special society stories or trend profiles in the *Times*. *New York* magazine. *The New Yorker* for ads. *Women's Wear Daily*. (You can get it on the stand in the St. Regis or at many stands around the middle East Side.) It has a column called "Eye" which is very spicy, if you consider "who ate where" spice. They have keys for restaurants. Like "Restaurant X" is La Grenouille. If you read the above, you'll be briefed. If you want to be prebriefed, subscribe to *Women's Wear Daily* by mail. Eugenia Sheppard's column has an "Around the Town" section which also does the who-is-where *shtick*.

New York has the sloppiest looking cops of

any major city in the world. They've all got Third Avenue fever with sideburns and droopy moustaches and uniforms to match. But all-in-all they're pretty good cops, counting the provocations of cop life in New York. They're not too polite, but they mean no harm. Most New Yorkers have very little respect for other New Yorkers. Why should the cops be different?

Taxi drivers. Ah, taxi drivers. They used to be unbelievably rude. But since their fares keep getting raised, they've turned half polite. Don't gab with them, though. They're usually bores.

Things that sound good but ain't: New York Athletic Club. It has great facilities but so-so membership. The Waldorf. The Rainbow Room. It has never come back as an "in" place. Tavern on the Green. Top of the Sixes Restaurant at 666 Fifth Avenue. Westchester County. Long Island, which sounds Fitzgerald snazzy but is actually suburbia-slobovia, if it's near the city. It means Cedarhurst, Freeport, etc., and they are by no means society country. *Any* suburban area within commuting distance (including New Jersey) is *very* suburban.

You can gently raise your eyebrow at the above addresses and poo-poo them without making a major error. Of course, if you raise your eyebrow and offend your best business prospect, you've made a *big* error, so raise your eyebrow in private or with other similarly inclined eyebrow raisers. I just wanted to give you a little looking-down-upon material, so if someone invites you to dinner in Mamaroneck or tells you he stays at the Waldorf (*not* the Towers) or invites you to lunch at the N.Y.A.C., you know where *you* stand and where *he* stands.

Remember what I've told you, keep lots of

tip money handy, and put some "in" New Yorkers
under obligation whenever they visit your city.
After all, isn't it worth dinner for four in Chicago
to see the inside of El Morocco?

Well, isn't it?

Global Tycoonery

After a few postwars years of "Who needs it? We're doing fine right here in the l'il ole U.S.A.," there's hardly a company today, large or small, that isn't involved in or talking about doing business abroad. Nice commuter types from Scarsdale or Sausalito or Shaker Heights suddenly find themselves getting passport photos, wondering if they need typhoid shots, and worrying about what you tip a bellboy in Frankfurt.

Chances are the first two countries you'll go to on business will be Britain and Japan—the former because Britain is the gateway to Europe and the latter because the rest of Asia at the moment seems only a gateway to Japan. Chances are, too, that you're liable to make a fool of yourself in both countries, sometime or other, not because you're the first American to get there, but because you're the last American to get there. Before you came a horde of other U.S. business blokes who have already learned the ropes (or who have *not* learned the ropes and are *still* making fools of themselves).

But a boo-boo now and then never devastated anyone. Nor do you have to practice toe-touching bows for Japan or locate a stiff hat for England before you board the plane. Business people all over the world are pretty much the same. A hangover gets things out of focus for them just as it does for us and a big, unexpected order makes the world look just as beautiful. Don't worry, you'll relate.

But there *are* some differences in the daily routine. It's like some guys who shave before they shower and others who shower before they shave. If they try to change the appointed order of things, they miss the 8:10 train and spend all day hating themselves. What I'll try to do here is give you an idea of what the routine is like over there, so you won't be thrown.

The main trick is to do things with *style* when you're abroad, remembering, however, that their style should not be *your* style. For instance, there is no American who looks more foolish to the British than one who tries to be "Britannic." An hour after he checks into his London hotel he "cawn't" remember his way to Oxford Street and tells the head porter "Cheerio!" Don't. Don't handkiss in Vienna, click your heels in Düsseldorf, bow deeply in Kyoto. It's not your style, Chester. Recognize their ways so you won't be too startled by them. Then stay your own good, old American self.

Traveling to England

Landing at Heathrow Airport is a pleasure. The customs procedure in London is the easiest in the world—no fuss, no growls, no bullying. Just politeness. And skycaps (porters) are *available*, able, and once more, polite. A fifty-pence tip is generous, but it's worth it.

Where do you get the British coins? You should always, when you travel abroad, have some coins ready by exchanging a few dollars into foreign coinage at the U.S. airport. This also allows you to play with the money on the way over, to make it as familiar to you as nickels, dimes, quarters, and dollars.

If you do get a long face here and there when tipping in England, it's because many tippees still aren't used to their relatively new decimal system. Don't let it ail you. Just thank heaven and the British authorities for having freed mankind from the horror of twelve pence to the shilling and twenty shillings to the pound. Funny thing, by the way: there are equivalent-looking coins in most countries, a *sort* of a dime everywhere, and a *sort* of a quarter. They not only look like our coins, they have similar tip value. In Britain, the ten-pence coin is like our quarter and will serve nicely in most tip situations. But stop thinking of pound notes as dollars; they're worth more than twice as much.

Where to stay in London? My advice: choose one of the seven top hotels—Claridge's, the Dorchester, the Connaught, the Savoy, the Ritz, the Barclay, or Grosvenor House. It doesn't really cost that much more, maybe ten dollars a day. But it makes a big difference. They are wonderful, comfortable hotels, and they'll make you *feel* good. And they carry prestige. Your British associates and clients can't help but be favorably impressed. It's *nice* to be able to say, "Call me at Claridge's." Or to write a note to a London hostess on Connaught stationery. (Sending flowers with your note? Flowers are inexpensive and beautiful in London, and any nearby florist will bill your hotel. The porter will handle it—*if* it's a first-class hotel. *All* London florists are first class.)

The porter is a very important man to all visitors. British hotels (in fact, nearly all European hotels, except those few, alas, which have adopted the American style) are run by the desk and hall porter system, in a sort of church and state division of authority. Matters of money and rooms are handled by the desk. The hall porter takes care of all the rest. You want a reservation for the theatre? Porter. Want to fly to Munich? Porter. Want to order something from a shop and have it sent to your room? Porter. You're going to the bar and are expecting a date? Porter. Hotel phone operators automatically check with the porter if your room doesn't answer; leave instructions with him concerning your whereabouts, if you choose to have your whereabouts known. He'll have things wrapped and mailed for you. He'll send up the morning papers. He'll find you chauffeurs and sun lamps and anything else that's legal. Tip him. For saint's sake, tip him! Put him on a *retainer*! This is beyond the 15 percent that will be tacked onto your bill for "service," the tips you don't have to give.

If you arrive at your hotel on a weekday morning, you'll probably start your stay by telephoning for appointments. Very few British hotels have automated phones. You'll depend on the operator. If she wants to call you back after you've given her the number, don't fight her. She will. If it takes her awhile, it's because your number is "engaged." Also, when she cuts the connection at the end of your call, it will cause your phone to ring once. Get used to it, so you don't pick up the phone to ask what she wants.* If you have a lot of phoning to do and want the utmost cooperation, the best thing is to find out where the hotel switchboard is and drop by with a pound note in a discreet envelope. Currency in envelopes always works wonders, all over Europe. In New York it is not certain that anything works wonders any more.

If you want to call your office in the States, by the way, the only convenient time you can do it for most American cities is in the late afternoon. A call placed at 5 P.M. in London will reach New York just before lunchtime. If it's Los Angeles you must call, you'll have to do it at cocktail-dinner time, about 7 or 8 in the evening, which is a nuisance. What's more, telephone traffic at that hour is very often murderous. So unless it's an absolute *must* that you phone, use the old cable. The hotel

---

* In England, at the end of a phone call you "ring off," literally. Also "calling an extension" is "ringing through."

porter—*of course*—will send it for you. Just be sure your room has cable forms. And your stateside office can cable you, at length, cheaply. They don't need to send a night-letter cable unless they're forwarding a four-page legal document. Of course, you can command someone from your office to get up at an ungodly hour to phone *you* at *your* convenience, but if you are a benevolent boss, let them cable. I have found IT&T to be best from the States and RCA Communications excellent from Britain.

When it comes time to leave the hotel for an appointment, you may well decide to hire a rental car, with chauffeur. (The porter will arrange it all, as we've said.) These chauffeurs are marvelous, all carefully uniformed with a sort of noble cockade on the fronts of their hats as if they were wearing your livery, even as the Duke's footmen and gardeners wear his. They know their town and they can park and wait for you, a particular blessing in London, where cabs are harder to come by than in New York.

London taxi drivers, if you can't afford the chauffeur, are quite like big-city taxi men anywhere. They are experts on everything and not especially servile. But London taxis are *clean* and you are expected to *use* the ashtray and not the floor for your ashes and stubs. You give a London cabby the address *before* you get into the cab and you pay him *after* you get out, the way they did it in old-time American movies. At night, cabs which are free have their signs lit, same as in New York. (Why do the British drive on the left?—which you'd damn well better get used to fast when you cross the street. It's tradition. It's the side on which you mount a horse.)

At your hotel, a taxi will of course be flagged by the doorman—or commissionaire as he is called in England. You give the address to him and he passes it along to the cab driver. It gives the man something to do, makes him feel wanted. English commissionaires are usually retired regular army noncoms or navy petty officers. They wear their campaign ribbons and are rather military, saluting hotel guests in an off-hand, top-kick-to-C.O. manner. Your conversation with him is likely to go something like this:

> You (to Doorman): "Morning."
> Doorman: "Sah . . ."
> You (pointing to the grey sky): "Gonna rain?"
> Doorman: "Oh, don't think so, sah. Bit of dew, y'know."
> (It starts to pour . . . buckets. Taxi pulls up. Doorman raises umbrella for you. You tell him "35 Regent Street." Doorman opens cab door for you. You give him ten pence.)
> Doorman (to you): "Mind your head, sah." (to taxi driver): "35 Regent Street." (back to you as water covers the taxi window in sheets): "Sah . . ." (and this time you get the salute).

This little dialogue illustrates another important point about Britain. All those "Sir"s. No matter how many times you hear it's over, don't you believe it. The caste system lives on in some ways, even if not in others. It's very much alive in hotels. There are those who serve and those who are served, and they are *not* equals. But, having your station in life, there is no shame in serving; rather, it is a calling that deserves respect. And it would be rude to treat those who serve you with anything but respect.

In Britain, it is therefore necessary to become accustomed to making requests rather than commands. "Would you mind . . .?" "Could I ask you to . . . ?" "When you have a chance, would you . . . ?" These are your obligations in return for those "Sir"s. The way to get along in Britain is to begin with courtesy on *your* part, and then your waiter will say, "Thank you, sir" even before he has been tipped. The policeman—call him "constable"—will call you "sir" when you ask directions. These are rituals, signal buttons which set well-oiled machinery in motion. The conversation with the doorman was like that: a naturally respectful exchange, but with a definite rule for each. (Don't *you* call *them* "Sir," unless you are having tea with Prince Phillip or dining with your friend's father.) This whole server-served routine becomes natural after a couple of days. In fact, the danger is that you'll try to fall into the role of English gentry and sound like Lord Tewksbury on his way to the hunt. Just stay American, Marvin.

There are other "sirs" in England, of course, the honorable kind. And it does get confusing, because here's one man called "Sir something-or-other" who is a venerable codger you've heard began life as a coal miner, and here's another "Sir something-or-other" who is a snot-nosed kid who has to ask permission to meet you for lunch.

Well, to be brief about it, there are "Sirs" who have earned the honorific. They are called "Knights." It's a medium-big-size reward for earning Brownie points and it gets hung on lawyers (O.K., "barristers") when they've lived long and useful lives, on doctors who have operated on the best of Britain, on architects who have won commissions worldwide, and on investment bankers who have built financial empires bringing glory to the pound and the queen and so on. Even (shudder) actors make it, when their name is Olivier. When they are real bigwigs, they usually end up with what is known as a "Life Peerage," meaning they are referred to as "Lord something-or-other," but they can't hand the title on to their kids. The wives of both "earned" Sirs and Lords are called Lady, which, for many fellows, is a persuasive reason to struggle for the title. Behind many a future Sir or Lord pushes a future Lady.

Then there are the Baronets, who have inherited their "Sirs." It's the lowest form of *hereditary* title. They themselves may have done absolutely nothing worthwhile in their lives other than having chosen their parents wisely. And then there are the various forms of inherited Lords, from Viscount up through Earl. All their wives are Ladies, too. Lord is a kind of catch-all title for anything above Viscount and this side of Duke. They are automatically members of the House of Lords, of course, so they do at least have some kind of job. Lords, by the way, just sign their *last* names; so if you get a letter signed "Bradham," and that's all, he's really Lord Bradham. Sirs will sign their whole name and Baronets will usually have "Bart." after their name, so you know they didn't really earn it.

How to address them? No, no, you do need to know, because titled types are all over business offices. It's not really very complicated. You call the Knights and Baronets "Sir Charles" or "Sir Oliver"—if their names happen to be Charles and Oliver, naturally—and their wives Lady Miller or

Lady Goldstein, if those are their last names. You call a Lord "Lord Walker" and his wife "Lady Walker." You never call him "Your Lordship" or "Milord." That's what his butler calls him, or the maitre d' at his club.

Big-time lawyers usually get to be "Q.C." or "K.C.," meaning Queen's Counsel or King's Counsel. Now that there's a Queen, it's Q.C., of course. But once Prince Charlie gets there, it'll be the other kind. Anyway, when you see Q.C. behind a lawyer's name, your bill will be, well, *heavy*.

About lawyers in Britain. There are barristers and solicitors. The barristers wear those wig things and appear in court to *try* cases. The solicitors do all the slavish work back at the office. Chances are that you'll only be involved with solicitors, because once you get involved with the Barrister boys, you'd better watch your tail. When one of those birds gets up to address the court and the judge— "M'Lud ..." ("My Lord" in barrister lingo)—you're in some sort of grave trouble. Besides, you can't hire a barrister. Only a solicitor can. Sort of like the family doctor bringing in the proctologist. (Well not quite like that.)

Accountants are called Chartered Accountants.

British businessmen quite often speak to each other by last name. "I say, Miller ..." is perfectly okay. Or "Dear Miller" at the top of a letter. It's the way they learned to address their social equals in private school and rather a compliment should they speak so to you. Conversely, they are very punctilious about addressing very senior servants, such as beloved old chauffeurs or the maitre d' at their clubs, as *Mister* Miller. It may sound strange to you to get into a club and hear a semistranger (you've met him three or four times) greet you by saying, "Hello, Murchison," and then hear him turn to the club maitre d' and say, "Mr. Grudge, there are two of us for lunch."

Many British business letters leave off the top line, so that the writer can *hand* write "Dear Tom" or—for closer friends—"My dear Tom." They also use, with business friends, the form "As ever" at the bottom, rather than our usual "Sincerely."

About using "Esquire" (Esq.) in addressing a letter. In America only lawyers use it to pat each other on the back. It is fading fast with some British firms who do frequent business with Americans. They usually address us "Yanks" as "Mr.," as we do, and sometimes they even accept letters addressed to "Mr." without visible flushing of the face. But in personal correspondence "Esq." is used quite freely; there's still a bunch of fellows who'd be insulted if you were to call them Mr. Thomas Ludlow instead of Thomas Ludlow, Esq. As an American, you're forgiven. But if they write *you* a personal letter without the use of Esq., you have my permission to be *furious*. Go ahead, work yourself into a lather. You have been snubbed.

Unfamiliar word usage may trouble you at first. The British, just like us, for example, will talk of "going to Europe." But to them it means crossing the Channel. In the old days they spoke of "the Continent" and things being "continental" (meaning not good and honest and clean, meaning not *British*). But since the advent of the Common Market, Britishers speak of "Europe" just as we do. Except they don't include *themselves*.

As for the word "English," don't make the super boo-boo of calling people English when they're not. They will indignantly tell you that they're Scottish or Welsh or Irish. Same deal here in the U.S. If an Englishman were to arrive and tell a feller in Atlanta, "You Yankees are a strange breed . . . ," he'd get himself flattened. Correct term for any one of the species is "British." Correct term for anything from up there, north of the border, is "Scottish." "Scotch" is whisky (spelled without the "e" over there). Although when you say whisky in Britain, it's Scotch, of course, of course, *of course*!

For those of you who are Jewish (don't be upset now), some people in England don't consider *Jewish* to be *English*, even if a Jewish family has lived in England since Cromwell was a pup. They're *British*, of course, and there's no slur intended. It's not a matter of anti-Semitism. It's just that antecedents are taken seriously in Britain, and you're English or Scottish or Jewish or Welsh and proud of it. *All*, in any case, are members of the U.K. (United Kingdom—Britain with Northern Ireland thrown in). *All* are subjects of the Queen.

Accents. Those devils. For a while it was all very simple. All middle upper-class and upper-class people spoke like David Niven. It informed all that one had gone to a very good old school. Everyone below that social stratum spoke with a regional accent—be it Cockney or Lancashire or Cornwall —and they sounded nothing like David Niven. (Except the Scots. They always spoke with a burr or were free to speak with a burr. They have always sounded like Sean Connery.)

Now things are changing. People who used to speak like David Niven are beginning to sound like David Frost, which is quite different. It has become a bit more fashionable to sound, well, working-class. Darndest thing is that it's hard to tell. Fellow in the bar speaks like Niven. One says, "Aha . . . a Peer of the Realm." And of course he is. Other fellow in the bar sounds like Frost and one says, "Aha . . . working-class self-made success," and then he also turns out to be a Peer of the Realm. And what's more his peerage is older than the Niven-type's. Second fellow might be a working Lord, an assistant account executive in an agency, who wants to make everyone around him feel comfy-cozy so they won't accuse him of waving his Eton tie. Man-of-the-people, you know.

And that word "school." In Britain it means *school*, not university. I realize our own universities often teach high school subjects and are really "schools." But *their* universities are just that —universities. Almost what we call graduate schools. What's more, in Britain it matters much more (either for snobbery or antisnobbery) where you went from the age of eight to seventeen than what happens to you afterward. So if you ask a Britisher where he went to school, he might say "Eton" or "Harrow" or "Chester Secondary" (which ain't Eton or Harrow by a long shot), but he won't spill his college. Most British business fellows don't go to university, unless they wish to become accountants or lawyers or engineers. Straight from Harrow into a bank.

Which brings one to the subject of Public Schools. A Public School in Britain is a very *private* school. The name "Public" came about hundreds of years ago because many rich kids were privately tutored at home. So to send a kid to school was in a sense, sending him to *public* tutors, there to join all the other aristocratic moppets. Nowadays, the Public Schools are under a bit of attack. Britain, since the World War II, has had several outbreaks of guilt about the upper classes. The Public Schools have quieted matters somewhat by opening their doors to more working-class kids, giving many scholarships in the process.

Anyway, despite all the yelling, most of the top dogs in British business are still Public-School boys ("Old Boys," as they're called on the inside), because the British Public Schools are so gosh darn *good*. They are superior schools, that's all. They teach superbly, far better than most of the world's private schools and without turning the kids into bookworms (the way the French and the Germans do). No wonder the British business establishment still recruits from the Public Schools. Today it's pretty tough for a British kid to slide through any one of the ten or twelve top schools on family connection or title. If he botches things up, he'll be bounced on his betitled duff.

Now, with all that preliminary background out of the way, we are ready to do business with the English. You should enjoy it. Forget that stuff about traditional reserve. Just don't fall all over an Englishman or call him by his first name right off the bat, and you'll usually find a warm conviviality. Given the choice of an air-travel companion, I'll take the British. The French are super stuffy. The Germans have little to say, beyond business matters—which, let's face it, is very often true of the American exec as well.

British businessmen dress conservatively; all that talk about Carnaby Street has never meant much in Establishment circles. So don't think you'll be out of it unless you have an Edwardian velvet suit. Stick to a dark suit, neatly striped shirt, discreet tie. They may forgive your long side-burns.

As for titles within corporations, the equivalent of our president or chief operating officer is managing director. Chairman in England is the counterpart of our chairman of the board. British boards tend to be harder-working and more involved than ours; they are not just a group whose advice is solicited now and then. Boards really decide things over there. Stockholders are usually called shareholders, an appellation one seldom hears in this country.

British executives are blessed in one way: British secretaries are *marvels*. You can confide in them, like telling them you've got to catch a plane and you need a quick call back. If their boss doesn't want to talk to you, you'll be let down so gently you'll feel braced and secure anyway. British secretaries are that way, which is one reason they are in demand everywhere worldwide.

Forget what you've heard about food in Britain being so-so. If you're told you'll be lunching in the company's executive dining room, don't fret; many major British companies have fine kitchens. And the restaurants in London are excellent. The British businessman is extremely knowledgeable about food and wines—and I don't mean just the ports and clarets we know about from English detective stories. They know their Burgundies and Moselles, the lot.

If your host takes you to his club, it's rather a high compliment to you. The majority of British businessmen aren't all that socially secure and have usually moved heaven and earth to get admitted to their club. (One lad I know, when told that he had been blackballed, asked, "How many black balls?" His crestfallen sponsor said, "Have you ever seen a jar of caviar?") But remember one thing: at British clubs, particularly the London clubs of the more venerable sort, there are fairly strict rules about not discussing business over lunch. You'll have to check your briefcase downstairs. You'll probably be discussing business in any case—after all, no one is going to bug your table—but it wouldn't "do at all" to have business papers on the table, and your host, the member, would get a stiffish reprimand from the house committee should the infraction be noted. You have to check your briefcase with your coat. Also note that you cannot smoke at lunch in good clubs —only after 2:30 P.M. *Beastly* sorry!

It would be a pity, though, if all you ever did discuss were business, for the British businessman is generally broadly educated and can talk far and beyond business and golf. They are politically bright and usually well-read. They can talk about manners, mores, plays, novels, what have you. And they *love* to gossip!

One caveat when conversing with the British: there exists a certain attitude, arising out of the country's comparative demise as a Super Power, which can cause some uncomfortable moments. They suffer, really, from a mild form of paranoia about it all and are very sensitive, even testy, when they suspect others are bragging about their superiority or putting them down. And they can, as a corollary, be somewhat dogmatic concerning those areas in which they believe they are still top dog. This will often take the form of their making statements and then asking you to agree, because to them the conclusion is foregone. They'll say, "But

then you people hate our red tape, don't you?",
meaning they consider us slightly slovenly, while
everything British, they feel, is very precise. Or,
they'll say, "But then we mustn't rush things over
here, must we?", meaning that Americans stumble
hastily and carelessly into decisions.

It's really quite harmless, this need for a bit of
self-assertion. But if your dander does rise, cool it;
wait for your moment and then give it back to
them. For example, if the service is interminably
long at a restaurant, you tell them, "We mustn't
rush things over here, must we?" For God's sake,
grin while you say it, and all will be well. After the
initial startled look, they'll guffaw. The British are
very fair; they do indeed have a marvelous sense
of humor, and they are really very good-natured.
The only time you will see a loss of temper in
Britain is when someone thinks he's been unfairly
treated by a maitre d' or a taxi driver or a train
conductor or something of that sort. Otherwise, all
should be calm during your stay. And a jolly good
stay it will be; you have Robert Morley's and my
promise!

Traveling on the Continent

For those of you who are first-time travelers (abject apologies to all others who are super globetrotters), being on the Continent means you are now through speaking English. That may seem like a pretty stupid and self-evident thing to say, but you'd be surprised how many upright American business fellers don't really, but *really*, realize they're in a foreign country until they arrive someplace where they can't ask for the men's room or make a phone call. And that can happen the moment you get to the airport.

Therefore, get one of those little pocket guides and brief yourself with a few rudimentaries, such as "skycap" and "taxi" and "How much?" And find out the real name for your hotel. For instance, you're staying at a hotel called the Imperial in some French town. To the French, it ain't the Imperial (*im-pee-re-al*); to them it's the *am-pay-ree-ahl*. If you want to get there, you'd better be able to say it their way.

And don't let anyone give you the old saw about "everyone speaking English." The hell they do. They may understand some *English*, but not Tulsa-Oklahoma-American, and even if they do know English, they may not feel like speaking it the week *you're* there because of something Kissinger did the day before or something their newspapers wrote that morning. This is particularly true in France. The French tend to hate all foreigners on principle. The French government, fully aware of this, has launched various campaigns trying to cajole Frenchmen into rudimentary civility. (The Swiss may not *like* you, but at least they're smart enough to be civil.)

All in all, however, despite years of America getting blasted by European newspapers and politicians, most Europeans are sort of fond of Americans. It's amazing—and damn satisfying—to realize how much goodwill we still generate.

Experienced traveler or not, and even if you know the language, I strongly urge that you prepare and keep preparing for each trip. Use all the "naive" tools for preparation, such as travel guides, phrase dictionaries, maps, etc. I travel unendingly, but I pick up every publication I can get, even about countries I know like the back of my hand. There is invariably something to learn. Particularly from maps. It's a great source of joy to be able to zing some taxi driver because you know his city's geography almost as well as he does.

Also, get to know the currency. There's no need to feel foolish because you can't hand out a correct tip or get correct change for a purchase. And don't try to tip *their* way. Tip *your* way. If you would have given a New York hackie a quarter tip, hand out the exact equivalent in francs or lire to his European counterpart. In restaurants, despite the 15 percent or so which is added to the check, the maitre d' in Rome is the same old maitre d' you would have tipped in New York or Los Angeles or Chicago. Tip him!

A word about traveling on the Continent. For most Americans, train travel, long-distance train travel, is a matter of history, as far in the past as surreys with fringes on the top. But in Europe there are still superb trains, and, if you are not absolutely *crushed* for time, use overnight trains. They are romantic and tasteful and the food is superior and you'll be able to indulge in all of your Bond-Coward-Maugham fantasies. ("I had no sooner settled in my compartment than I saw her through the glass sliding door. She was obviously on her way to the bar car. The porter palmed my 10,000-lire note and provided her name. . . .")

Hotel life all over the Continent, as in England, is centered around the hall porter, but now he'll probably be called a concierge. Put yourself into his hands. Whenever you see the frock coat with the crossed keys (this is pretty much the universal signal for the concierge and his chief assistants), bribe him and leave everything to his care.

In continental hotels you don't call up for valet or room service, by the way. There are usually little bell-buttons on your night table with little pictures in case you can't read the language. I mean, what's "valet" in French?

Be sure to wrap yourself in your towel when room-service waiters or maids knock on the door. They come right in. Boom. Just like that. Without waiting for you to say O.K. Sure, sometimes they're pretty girls. But sometimes they're ugly men. So wrap up.

Yes, you can leave your shoes outside the door to your room for overnight polishing, but it won't make much difference. No one in Europe knows how to shine shoes. Your loafers will be returned in the morning looking like they've been massaged with sour cream.

If you're an electric razor fan, remember that your razor and European current and plugs might not agree. Go to your neighborhood hardware shop and get a converter and converter plugs.

As for dress, businessmen in France are fairly formal, so bring fairly formal clothes if you're heading for Paris. It's quite difficult in America (and these days even in Britain) to judge business-men by their apparel. But not in France. They still believe that white shirts, dark suits, and dark ties are the mark of the reliable man. ("*Un homme sérieux*" is their way of saying a sound, solid, dependable citizen; it has nothing to do with "seri-ous." In fact, many *hommes sérieux* keep some pretty kicky mistresses, and that ain't serious—except to their wives.)

One of the curious things is that in many parts of Europe, though mainly in Italy and France, the "gentry" try to look like old-time Brit-ish aristocrats with lots of chalk-stripes and high side-vents and tweedy country suits *mit* leather elbow patches. So if you arrive on the European Continent wearing your fake British-American clothes, you'll be quite okay in France and Italy. As for the so-called "French" look or "Italian" look, I have yet to discover either one. Most of the things which are marked down as "typically French" or "typically Italian" are really imitation "uppah-clawss" British: high armholes and raised waistlines and long side-vents and all.

Only thing is the British don't dress that way anymore, except for a few recluse squire types in the Counties or secondhand-Bentley salesmen in the dowdier parts of London.

Now each country has its own set of guest manners. For instance, in Sweden one sends flowers to one's hostess *before* one gets to her home. In England one usually sends the "thank-you" posies afterwards. In Spain you eat at ungodly late hours and usually in all-male company. In France you eat earlier. There's no sense in trying to compile a guest-guide here. Best thing to do is ask a local who seems to have reasonable manners. (Don't ask the taxi driver. He won't know. Anymore than he would in New York.)

Most expatriates are pretty good about that sort of thing, too. So if you know an American fellow who's lived in Rome or London or Copenhagen for a while, ask him. Trouble with most American expatriates is that usually they turn out to be more British than the British, more Greek than the Greeks, etc. But that'll be to your advantage, because the expatriate businessman is usually the very heart and soul of good local manners.

Finally, since this book has to do with image, the making of the image, the losing of the image, the right image, the wrong image, etc., let me get to the subject of the *self*-image which an American should have.

Wrong: To feel like a country bumpkin, visiting the cradle of civilization. It just ain't so. It's many, many, many generations since Americans were funny colonials living across the wide Atlantic, who married off their rich daughters to the impoverished European gentry, who, in turn, taught Americans how to use which fork in which hand. Bunk. *Super* bunk. Today's Americans are probably the most sophisticated people in the world. We're the most avant-garde, the most adventuresome, the hardest to please. That's because for decades we've been the wealthiest and that (happily or unhappily) is the basis for much of our sophistication. Playwrights and painters, musicians and sculptors, polo players and Rolls Royce salesmen all drift in the general direction of *money*. Any ten blocks of New York (East Side), Chicago (North Side), Los Angeles (Beverly Hills Side) or, for that matter Dallas, can produce more art collectors, expensive cars, musicians, whores, yachts, homosexuals, fine cuisine, tasteful homes, great hostesses, and civilized hosts than many entire European countries can. Fact is that most Palm Beach yachts are owned. Most Cannes yachts are chartered.

So *never* let anyone *ever* hand you any nonsense about the "uncivilized" American. (The British gave up a while back. They have now appointed the Australians as the butt of that stuff.)

Also understand that the European image of us is, to a certain degree, one romantically fabricated through years of films and, more recently, TV series. They often cannot quite reconcile the Gary Cooper cowboy or Fred Astaire playboy with the visitor from the States. So they overreact by attempting to snub.

Take full assurance from the fact that New York *far* outglosses Paris, London, and Rome; that Palm Beach is a jewel compared with Europe's finest beach resorts; that for the theater aficionados (of whom I'm not one) New York's is head and shoulders above European theater (except, and not always, for London).

But once you have reinforced yourself, don't go overboard. Don't get snotty, Chester!

Traveling to Japan

Japan is the most punctual country in the world. You'll be expected to be exactly on time for all meetings. Long schedules are prepared ahead of time. You'll get your copy. If you're early, it doesn't matter. They'll still stick to the original time brackets. They have an agenda of subjects to be covered and so many days to complete the agenda and by prescheduling they manage to cover all subjects. If you change anything in the schedule, you have caused the following problem: Japanese businesses are run by teams of specialists, and chances are that only the people who are directly involved in a given subject will attend a specific meeting. Therefore, out there, poised to jump, is a fellow who knows that *his* subject will be covered at 8:13 A.M. (yes, they start work early in Japan). And if you start his subject at 8:01 A.M., he's liable not to be there, because he is still in his previous meeting or having a second cup in the coffee shop. The way the Japanese businessman stays efficient is by sticking to his schedule.

The card routine. When first meeting a new face, Japanese businessmen hand each other a business card. It's a bit of a ceremonial accompanied by bows and the muttering of one's own name. It

originated, one assumes, with the fact that there
are vast numbers of Japanese families with the
same name. (You think there are a lot of Smiths in
the Chicago phone book? You ought to know how
many Suzukis or Yamamotos there are in the
Osaka phone book.) So the Japanese businessman,
who *never* uses the other fellow's first name (even
if they went to grade school with each other),
would be completely befuddled without a card
which says: "K. Suzuki, Manager, Marketing Sub-
department, Fuji Coal Company, Osaka." He now
becomes, in the mind of the card recipient, "The
Fuji Coal Marketing Suzuki from Osaka," so that
he does not get him confused with the N. Suzuki
who is the advertising manager at Fuji or the
L. Suzuki who is the president of a rival coal company in Nagoya.

They don't use first names? Then how in
Hades do they ever get to be chummy? How do
they slap each other on the back at the end of the
day over a glass of booze or trade romantic tales on
the golf courses, huh? They have their ways. They
condense the first name and slur the word *san*,
which means "Mr." but is tacked on after a Japanese name. A man called Kakiuchi, for instance,
who is normally *Kakiuchi-san*, becomes *Kek-san*
when you yell at him in a friendly way across an
airport lobby because your plane is leaving and
he's rushing over from the men's room. It's the
Japanese equivalent of "For Chrissake, Mike, get
your butt moving!"

Do you hand out cards? Yes. Why not. Bring
plenty. They go fast when you hand out six or
eight a meeting. But don't attempt the Japanese
bow, except in a *slight* way. In fact, most Japanese
businessmen will expect to shake hands with you,

and you'd be much better off greeting people as you do in America. Several Japanese friends have told me that they're—well, *suspicious*—of a foreigner who tries to act too Japanese.

Suggestion: You'll meet dozens of people all day long, all of whom have similar names. Take their cards, shove them into your left (okay, right) jacket pocket and at the end of the day, sort them all out and write yourself a who's who. Otherwise you'll be lost after three days. Also, you won't know who's boss and who ain't. Japanese corporations are divided and subdivided like no others, and the titles are not the same as ours. The basic difference between Japanese and American corporations is that second- and third-level managements are often not in the *decision* business. They are in the *recommendation* business. They will study and prepare and then recommend to a small, very senior elite, and it's the *top* boys who'll give the final okay. So there is often a time lag. But once a Japanese decision has been made, it gets followed through to the end. (Which is not always the case in the U.S.A.)

The big title in Japan is director, and even bigger is executive director (with various grades, such as senior executive director). They are the Japanese versions of our vice-president, senior vice-president, executive vice-president, etc. The really *super* big boys above them do indeed have the titles of vice-president and president, but they are the equivalent of our chairman of the board, associate chairman and president. In Japan, vice-president is really super-duper-top-flight, whereas our own vice-presidents are often mass-produced. The Japanese equivalent of our veeps are the directors, get it?

Usually, a Japanese company has an executive board of sorts, and that's "where it's really at." When a man's title is *executive* director, he's a member of the *executive* board and therefore in on all the major decision-making; so he's more than the average director. Look for that word "executive" before the title. Anyway, it's all on the cards, or ask each corporation for its annual report. The whole hierarchy is usually spelled out. Don't let the word *sub*department fool you, either. It can be a very large department and the manager may be very strong. The same guy in an American firm would probably be called director of promotion or director of marketing or something equally commanding.

An odd side issue to the business-card exchange is that senior-senior Japanese executives have very small cards with very little information on them. The president of a major company may have a small card imprinted with his name and the name of his company. That's all. At a certain level of prominence, Japanese executives do not hand out cards. They are expected to be known. They also bow less effusively. There are bows and there are, well, bows. In Japan, as everywhere else—in fact, more than everywhere else—the boss is the boss.

Speaking of bosses, in Japan careers are slow to mature. Patience is essential. Senior executives usually have gray hair. The bright young hot shot is *not* part of the Japanese industrial scene. At least, not verbally. He may be a hot shot, but in a meeting with his seniors he shuts up until spoken to.

All Japanese are naturally courteous and like to make a good impression on foreign visitors; so even the president of a very major company will ask you to go through doors and into elevators ahead of him. Don't take your acceptance for granted. If you are a junior vice-president of your company and he is president of his, ask *him* to go ahead of *you*. In Japan the matter of *age* is still important, and you should treat him with the courtesy due to your elders. Forget the fact that your company may be bigger than his and that you may be the customer. Think of him as a friend of your father's. Come to think of it, chances are that his company is bigger than yours, anyway.

Japanese meetings are conducted in meeting rooms, not in offices. Japan is notoriously short of real estate and private offices are space wasters. Some surprisingly responsible executives in Japan, who would have slick offices in this country, have no private office. They function at a desk set in a large room, along with many other executives, like American newspaper offices or neighborhood banks. A few very senior executives have private offices. Still, even they usually greet you in meeting rooms, which are quite rigidly decorated. Two couches flank a long coffee table with two armchairs at each end. There will probably be extra chairs around the sides of the room for extra people, but usually the senior participants sit in the couches or armchairs.

Everyone in Japan smokes . . . lots. Tea is served, or soft drinks. The first few minutes are spent in courtesies. Since the meeting is usually prebriefed, you can approach the subject matter in reasonably short order, but you will often find that you are expected to present it as if there had been no previous briefing. Often the man speaking for the other side is not necessarily the boss. The top man may sit next to the speaker, listening. It's a gambit used by the older generation of Japanese executives. It gives them a sense of perspective and objectivity. Eventually they'll speak up, but at the beginning it's "listen and judge" time. You, as the American, won't be able to do so, but if you want to force the issue, you can always address the big boy directly. That'll involve him more rapidly.

Now to interpreters. You can take your six-week course at Berlitz and be great about ordering a *sushi* dinner or buying camera lenses on the Ginza, but don't try to talk business in Japanese or have a general conversation unless you are an absolute Japanese scholar. Japanese is a very, *very* subtle language and you may offend someone deeply by innocently conveying the wrong meaning. Sort of like a Japanese telling your wife that he reached his hotel at midnight but "could not get laid until 2 A.M.," when he really meant that he could not get to sleep until 2 A.M. From his point of view, what's wrong with "laid"? After all, it means "lie down" and therefore "sleep" doesn't it? The hell it does.

The great disappointment in Japan is that very few interpreters speak perfect English. And when they do speak perfect colloquial American, beware! Chances are that they're Nisei (born in the U.S.A.) or Japanese who spent all their school years in this country. They are therefore almost *foreigners* to the Japanese and are treated with suspicion. Or they may speak "poor" Japanese in the sense that they sound slovenly or slangy or even rude to the educated Japanese businessman.

The best *you* should count on from an interpreter is "Berlitz English." What *does* matter is how he says things in *Japanese*! You may have to spend a lot of effort conveying your meaning to your interpreter, but it's worth it if it comes out in pure and tactful Japanese. Be sure you ask your interpreter over and over if he understands your meaning. The Japanese have a great knack of saying "yes" when they don't really understand you, because they don't want to impose on you for further clarification. Have your interpreter explain to you what you are trying to get him to say. It matters that you control him before you release him. Also, avoid having him become embroiled in a conversation which you launched. There is the temptation for an interpreter to *speak for you*. The moment that your one sentence becomes an interchange between the interpreter and them, stop him. He may be getting you into hot water without meaning to.

Japanese is a very laborious language compared to modern-day American business talk. Don't get impatient. A simple question like "Could you tell me another way of getting it shipped?" may seem endless in the translation. Or a slang expression like "No thanks. I've had it," may throw your interpreter into a tailspin. He sits there asking himself "He's had what? When did he have it?" etc., etc. So make it clear. If you can't eat any more, for example, simply and clearly say, "Thank you, no. I have had enough to eat." Also, don't use any words of the moment, like "super" or "fabulous." Say "fine" or "very good" or "excellent."

The matter of "face." When you are really furious in a business discussion, don't let Japanese associates feel it. Never chew anyone out in front of others, even if you know he is at fault. Tell him that you know it isn't his fault and that there must have been a mistake in another department or an oversight by another division. Also, if you ask an embarrassing question ("I still don't get it. Why in hell didn't those parts get shipped on time?"), and he cannot answer, he will simply *not* answer. He will shrug and smile and go off on a tangent, but he won't address himself to your question. It's his way of stalling until he has the answer for you or has concocted a good excuse. Don't pursue the matter. Drop it. You won't gain by your persistence. The next day, at an unexpected moment, he'll suddenly give you a memo about that shipment—probably that his firm shipped on time, but that the American carrier goofed.

You'll also run across the "So sorry" syndrome. The Japanese apologize and smile while apologizing. Don't let it annoy you. An apology in Japan is a bit of self-punishment. In earlier days, when Japan was still an isolated island community with even stricter rules of social behavior, a man who said "I'm sorry" punished himself by openly admitting to a mistake. It's a lot milder self-castigation today, but the habit lingers on.

The Japanese business day is tense and terse and formal. The evening is there to relax and unbend. Business dinners can be fairly raucous in an all-male, almost boyishly innocent way. They are strictly *men* dinners, certainly never *family* dinners. The dames who sometimes appear, magically, are, well, *dames*. It's up to you if you want to or not. Nobody will hold it against you or blackmail you; nor do you have to feel you must prove your virility. The Japanese like self-control and display a high degree of admiration for men who keep themselves in check in every way: temper, booze, broads.

Japanese-style dining seems to be super worri-some to most first-time visitors and even to some old-timers. Understandably. It's as different (to us) as dining with a Kuwaiti oil sheik in his palace, or joining a genuine royal Hawaiian luau. You'll take off your shoes. So beware of "leaky" socks. You'll then be confronted with slippers which, chances are, will be too small for you. Use them with care. You can dump them the moment you sit down. The old Japanese "formal" way of sitting (on your heels) is rapidly disappearing. At the very beginning of a dinner, your host, if he is a bit old-fashioned, may still sit that way himself, a gesture of courtesy toward you. He will then get off his heels and sit loosely and invite you to do the same. When wearing Western clothes, Japanese men shed their jackets at dinner. It is quite accept-able, because business dining in Japan is always all male, except for waitresses and hired female "com-panions."

A formal Japanese geisha dinner—whatever you might think—is a bit boy-scouty. The geisha may press her hand on your (aching) knee as you sit cross-legged at the table, but she really doesn't mean it. She's just doing her very ceremonial best, and the hand on the knee is part of a hundreds-of-years-old tease routine. When the geishas dance and sing you must look at it as though you were watching an American hoedown. The Japanese are very fond of their folk stuff and enjoy it. We're apt to slough off ours, but maybe that's *our* loss.

About eating Japanese meals. Don't be so damn squeamish. Give it an honest try. Ask your dining neighbors about how you put what food on what. If the raw fish and such is just not your dish, at least you will know that at most of your lunches

Western food will be served. Japanese businessmen lunch on steaks and sandwiches, just as we do.

Most of them prefer whisky to Sake. Their whisky is Scotch. But you'll get a taste or two of sake, particularly if you do get invited to a geisha dinner. It's delicious, warm or cold. The correct toast is "*Campai*" (like "*Skol*," "Cheers," etc.). It is courteous to fill your neighbor's glass. He will pick it up and hold it while you are pouring. Do the same when he is pouring for you. When you have made very good friends—and this is truly a gesture of trust and liking—they will involve you in *Hempai*. In *Hempai* sessions, a man will come over to where you are sitting (on a pillow) and fill your glass. You will then finish it bottoms up, act as if you are emptying the last drop into your palm, hand it to him, and fill it for him. He will then finish it, act as if he is shaking the last drop into his palm, fill it up again, and hand the glass back to you. You will then finish it, etc., etc., etc. Timber!

There are a dozen of these little formalities which you can learn, but there's no sense trying to teach you them all here and now. Wait until you're there. Japanese love to teach their customs, and they're never, never bored telling you about Japan and Japanese manners and history. They are hesitant, however, to tell you about Japanese morals and mores, because they're very *private* people.

A classic example: Once, at Kabuki Theater in Tokyo, when I asked my highly educated Japanese host-companion (he was a university professor) if all the female impersonators (there are no actresses in Kabuki) are homosexual, I drew a blank. The gay male is absolute anathema to the average Japanese man; he is much more vehemently ostracized than in the West. Every gesture, every word in Japan must look and seem *male*. By the way, the Japanese gesture for "no" is hand and forearm moved laterally in front of one's face, but stiff wristed. (A limp wrist is, of course, a gesture of being "limp-wristed.")

There is still much of the Samurai, the ancient warrior, in each Japanese businessman. He admires the manly traits, such as punctuality, reliability, honesty, capacity for booze, prowess at sports, resilience, tenaciousness, endurance, and love of family and children. The Japanese are enormously proud of good scholarship, good athletic ability, and good manners among their kids. They will never brag, but, once given a chance, they will begin to talk. Bring your kids' photos. Japan is filled with doting pops. You might even bring your wife's photo.

And yet, face the fact that you may not get to see your business friend's home or family, at least not on your first trip and perhaps not on your fifth trip. That's the way it is. The Japanese are extremely shy about their homes and families. Furthermore, many of them commute long distances daily to the cities and do so via uncomfortably crowded trains. Chances are you'll be doing business in Tokyo or Osaka. Chances are they'll live an hour away.

What will you talk about during social hours? Certainly don't involve yourself in any rehash of the war. That would be stupid and pointless. But besides the usual family and cultural banter, you can certainly talk sports.

If you're a golfer, you're *in*.

If you're a tennis player, you're *in*.

If you're a skier, you're *in*.

If you're a bowler, you're *in*.

If you're a sailor, forget it. It's not a country with many facilities for the sort of boat loafing, sailing, fishing we're used to.

The Japanese have a great sense of humor. Ain't nothing "inscrutably Oriental" about them. Catch them in areas which they understand. Gags about golf (they are golf-*mad*) or baseball or expense accounts or wives or nonwives are fully understood. They love to laugh. Make the joke simple, though, because chances are ten to one it must be translated for you. Japanese have subtle and complicated wits but interpreting jokes is a tough business.

Japanese hostmanship is unending. You will receive gift after gift. Open and admire. But be sure to open carefully, without hurting the paper, because wrapping means a lot in Japan and it is part of the thought behind the gift. In turn, on your second trip, you may want to bring gifts for friends. Don't be too extravagant, but do be *thoughtful*. Japanese are very thoroughly educated, and they are great students, lifelong. A book about American history or art or architecture will be better received than an American tie. Nearly all Japanese executives are university graduates and ruthlessly well-read. In Germany you'll find a bunch of business guys who, like yourself, really can't remember when Charlemagne reigned or what the Council of Trent decided. Not in Japan. They know their own history and culture and they love to study ours. Realize that the man sitting opposite you might have been one of 20,000 students in a top university, who was chosen by his corporation in his junior year to become part of their future executive pool. He has been studying since the age of five, *hard*. It's ingrained.

The dinners and the gifts are fine, but after a while there's a tendency for foreigners to feel that Japanese business hosts *own* you. Every moment is taken up with business or entertainment. To repeat, they are enormously hospitable and kind. But we suggest that you sneak some spare time for yourself. Being alone on a Japanese street for the first time, separated from your hosts and the interpreter, is a bit like a student pilot's first solo flight. The further you get from the hotel, the more you wonder if you can find your way back. But it's worth it, in many ways, not the least of which is the matter of just being *alone*. Since very, very few visitors to Japan speak fluent Japanese, the constant flow of interpreted polite conversation is absolutely *draining*. It's like being in an eternal squash game, where you have to stay active and attentive. Never worry about being money-cheated during your "solo flights." The Japanese are very honest. Just hand out a bill, and they'll give you correct change.

By the way, in Japan there is no hotel or restaurant tipping in the American sense. They pack the tips into the bill, European style. However, you do hand out small coins, sort of courtesy tips, to bellboys and room service. Ask your Japanese friends. They'll tell you the "right" amount.

Japanese hotels are run much like American hotels, which is their misfortune. Just as in America, everything in a Japanese hotel concentrates around the reception desk—unlike the hall-porter system we've discussed in European hotels. Thereby, too, hangs a problem, because, just as in

the U.S., it's too darn much for one small group of
desk clerks to handle. It must be admitted that the
Japanese reception clerk is better than his average
American counterpart. Telephone operators are
quite good, provided you stick to the things they
have been taught, such as numbers and basic
sentences like "Room Service, please." If you go
off on benders like trying to find out what the
weather will be like, you're in trouble.

There are Western-style hotels and Japanese-
style hotels. Although the Marco Polo in you will
be tempted to try a Japanese-style hotel, don't!
They're wonderful hotels, but they'll just be too
strange for you. For instance, they rarely have
dressers or closets, and you'll end up literally living
out of your suitcase. Also, Japanese-style men's
rooms—and ladies' rooms—are different and you
have to be quite athletic to use them.

Western-style Japanese hotels have consoles
next to the bed which include everything from
radio to night light. The light is very necessary,
because Japan is earthquake country. It is much
more shaky and trembly than California, and when
you are awakened by your rolling room at 3 A.M.,
you will want a light, and quick. After centuries of
wooden houses which went up in centuries of
flames, the Japanese are very fire-hazard-happy and
have the best fire departments in the world. So you
won't find any ashtrays on your night table. When
they say "Don't smoke in bed," they *mean* it!

In every halfway decent Western-style Japanese hotel, you will get a *Yukata* or kimono-style
robe, allover printed with the hotel's symbol. They
give you a fresh one each evening. They're absolutely marvelous. You'll feel tempted to steal them.
You *will* steal them. You'll want to tell the desk

clerk, but if you're really larcenous, you won't. Either way, if you pack one, they'll usually charge you for it anyway. If you have any sense, you'll own four of them by the time you leave Japan.

One final dollop of advice: If you intend to go to Japan with any degree of frequency, say once a year, it would be a really good idea to pick up a book on Japanese history. I realize you don't want to play student-tourist, but Japan is different. Even the densest traveler to Britain has heard about Henry VIII and Good Queen Bess. But very few foreigners know anything at all about Japanese history and Japan *is* history! Every moment of every day you will bump into manners, morals, attitudes, meals, conditions which are planted in their history, like the "So sorry" thing I mentioned before. It's terribly important that until quite recently (120 years ago) Japan was locked up . . . tight. No foreigners, no interchange. So they developed a very unique set of attitudes which studying their past can help you understand. Also realize that this huge industrial complex is locked up in a physical area the size of California, along with 100 million people and a lot of uninhabitable mountains. No wonder things in Japan are a bit more regulated. Get a book and read it. Your visits will mean a lot more.

One Final Memo

I realize that telling people how to (or how *not* to) do things, as I've been doing in these pages, is a bit like playing leapfrog with a unicorn. You have to do it carefully. Yet, with all mature caution and considered moderation, you still have to tell things straight, even though in the process you are bound to dent a few vanities, make a few enemies, raise a few howls.

I don't mind the howls. I've been yelled at by salt-sprayed masters of the roisterous curse. I am at all times willing to assume that I am wrong as hell. But I usually find that the loudest howls arise when I have hit an unprotected posterior, leading me to believe that the howler was, in effect, caught with his pants down.

But if there is anything you have learned in the process of reading this book, and if you feel the lesson was useful, I am satisfied. In fact, go ahead, make it your own. What the heck—you don't even have to admit you read this book!